The SUPER Antioxidants

The SUPER Antioxidants

Why They Will Change the Face of Healthcare in the 21st Century

James F. Balch, M.D.

M. Evans and Company, Inc. | *New York*

M. Evans and Company, Inc.
216 East 49th Street
New York, New York 10017

Design and composition by John Reinhardt Book Design

Printed in the United States of America

ATTENTION:
Advice in this book must not be taken without the consultation of your personal physician. Please read the Author's Note on page xii.

Contents

This book is first dedicated to my compassionate and wise wife, Dr. Robin Young-Balch, who unceasingly encouraged me during the production of this book.

Also, to all those seekers of the truth who desire to maintain a sound state of health for themselves and their loved one.

And finally, to the many health care providers who will assist in the healing of the multitudes because of this work.

Introduction

Congratulations! I'm very proud of you. In my opinion, the single most important thing that you can do today is to learn more about your health. It's wise and prudent to be healthy. It's a wonderful thing when someone decides to take personal responsibility for the improvement of his or her health. This book will help you accomplish that. By picking up this book, you have taken the first small step toward improving the quality of your life by accepting responsibility for your health. In these pages you will find invaluable information which will help you accomplish that goal by assisting you in understanding a subject that is poorly understood, even by those in the medical profession: the importance of antioxidants in a health and preventive maintenance program.

This book will present a very interesting paradox to you: oxygen is essential for life, yet oxygen also contributes to your aging and death. It is a puzzle with which I have been dealing since illness struck my own household more than twenty years ago.

In the late 1970s, my wife and children became chronically ill and, despite my medical training and experience, I could not discover what was wrong with them. I took the traditional approach to seeking a cure for their illness, spending a vast amount of time and money on this endeavor. But, even with access to the best medical advice available, I could not discover the underlying cause of their problems. Finally, I realized that the traditional medical approach was not going to work in this instance.

Reluctantly, I approached an alternative physician and famous naturopath who suggested that the problem could be an allergy, a reaction to the foods my family was consuming. I was surprised when he asked me the question, "Do you think that it is what your family is eating that is making them sick?" But I was even *more* surprised when he added, "Did you know that the foods your family eats can make them well again?"

The simplicity of his words shocked and stunned me, but they also brought home the message that my family and I were becoming what we ate. At that time, this concept was foreign to me. I had never really been taught the fundamental truth that the body's health is linked directly to the nutrients we do or do not ingest, or that we could be poisoning our bodies with the very foods we are eating.

But, as I saw my wife and children get better and eventually become completely healed through dietary changes and supplementation, I vowed that this approach to health and healing would not go unexplored. It was then that my quest to understand alternative methods of healing began.

I quickly determined that the cornerstone of better health is the immune system and its integrity. Without a properly functioning "on board" defense system, the body is vulnerable to attack from a multitude of microbes (germs) and the ravages of free radicals (oxidants). Free radicals? No one had ever told me about free radicals. What are they? I soon learned that free radicals (oxidants) are countered by antioxidants. But what are antioxidants? Simply put, antioxidants are the "good guys" and free radicals (oxidants) are the "bad guys."

I had read many studies which provided overwhelming evidence that antioxidants curtail, prevent, and in some cases, cure many diseases. Gradually, I began to understand that the theories of disease that I had been taught in medical school were incomplete. Many of the disorders I dealt with frequently, such as cancer and heart disease, could not be explained by the germ theory I had been taught. There had to be more. As I investigated further, the big picture began to come into focus.

I found that alterations in the immune system were responsible for cancer and heart disease, the major killing diseases of our society. At the same time, I realized the importance of antioxidation in combating oxidative stress. This concept of "oxidative stress" through the reactive oxygen species (ROS)—the free radicals which damage our bodies—is an important factor in premature aging, disease, and death, and was unknown to me before I began my investigation.

In recent years, there has been a shift in the disease paradigm. Traditional modern medicine tells us that most diseases are caused by germs, and that in order to get well we must kill these germs. Toward that end, we use drugs, antibiotics, chemotherapy, radiation, and even surgery.

However, the school of thinking of which I have now become a part involves other forms of complementary healing arts that are not a part of the traditional medical practice. We are only now beginning to fully understand how disease results from an imbalance in the body and the chaos and disorder in the body function that is brought on by nutritional imbalance or "intoxication." In order to re-establish health, one needs to balance the body by working with it, not against it.

As a urological physician and surgeon for thirty-five years, I had followed a traditional course of treatment for my patients; however, I had become dissatisfied with many of the results of treating disorders that I confronted, particularly cancer of the urinary bladder and prostate. As I began complementing traditional surgical and treatment methods with nutritional supplementation and dietary change, I discovered that my patients were not only improving, many of them were being healed in an almost miraculous fashion! As a result, they were much happier than patients who underwent radical surgical procedures followed by chemotherapy and/or radiation.

I had never really considered myself a teacher, but in truth doctors are teachers, and I soon found that teaching patients better health through nutritional supplementation and dietary changes produced a healing that I had never before witnessed. It was truly an impressive thing. First, I found that any protocol of the healing art must be based on a foundation of solid *nutrition* and *diet* which leads to homeostasis (balance in the body).

Proper digestion and a properly functioning immune system are necessary to combat not only foreign bacteria, but also the internal effects of free radical damage. The *key* to the healing of the body is *balance and antioxidation.*

The second element I learned, and equally as important as the first, is that toxins must be eliminated from the body. Detoxification is an essential aspect of the body's healing process. Third, I determined that *moderation* is necessary to good health. Finally, it became apparent that any successful treatment must deal with *the whole body* The physical body is important, of course, but the soul and the spirit must be dealt with as well. The mind, emotions, and the very will of man and the stresses linked to everyday existence can cause serious disease.

What destroys the body? According to Steven C. Denk, author of the *New Health Resources Manual,* "it is diet and environmental factors which alter nutritional balances and homeostasis processes that ultimately lead to acidification and oxygen deprivation. Parallel to this is lymphatic stasis which potentiates the body's failure to remove trapped blood proteins and toxin buildup. It, in turn, runs parallel to overall bowel toxicity. These are the core factors which push the degenerative biological realities into gear that make you rot, and kick-starts the biochemical/electronic mechanisms which make you rust," Denk asserts. "When you talk specifics about something like food and what negatively impacts the body, we can list things like tea, coffee, [too much] alcohol, tobacco, soft drinks, drugs (both prescription and over-the-counter), too much salt, too much sugar, candy, cake, ice cream, pop with caffeine, high-fat content of food, too much cooked food, too much processed food, too much meat, yet basically these are the things that most of us are living on each day."

Simply, we are "rotting and rusting" to death because of the very things we do or do not eat, drink, or breathe. The good news is that this Rot-Rust Syndrome can be prevented, stopped, and reversed!

There is an ancient joke about a man who goes to the doctor and is told to give up just about everything he enjoys in life for his health. When the doctor tells him to quit drinking, smoking, keeping late hours, and eating rich foods, the man asks, "Doctor, if I do these things, will you guarantee that I will live to be 100 years old?" The doctor looks him straight in the eyes and said, "No, but I guarantee that it will *seem* like 100 years!"

Living a full, healthy life doesn't mean giving up everything which makes it worth living; however it does require that we make a commitment to wellness based on responsible decisions about nutrition and lifestyle. *Remember, you truly are what you eat.* If, by pointing you down the right path, this book helps you achieve the goal of a long and healthy life, then the time and energy required in writing this book will have been well spent.

I know you will agree with me that it is wise and prudent to maintain your good health, but, as you will see, there is much to know about staying well or, if you are sick, how to get well again. Your understanding of the principles of antioxidation and your use of the "good guy" antioxidants through diet and supplementation will go a long way toward assuring you perfect health. In my opinion, that should be the goal of any wise man or woman. I desire the very best for you in this, your most rewarding quest.

Here's to wishing you a long, prosperous and healthy life!

Author's Note

The information contained in this book is based upon the author's personal experiences and research, as well as in-depth medical, laboratory, and experimental research published by contemporary professionals throughout the world. All publications and Internet sources of information utilized in this book have been obtained from the public domain.

This book is not intended to be a substitute for consultation with your personal physician and/or health care provider. The publisher, author, and/or experts specifically cited in this publication are not responsible for any consequences, direct or indirect, resulting from any reader's actions(s). All dosages listed are recommended ranges for healthy individuals, and each person's body type and tolerance levels(s) are calibrated differently. You, the reader, are instructed to consult with your personal physician prior to acting on any suggestions contained in this book. The purpose of this publication is to educate the reader as to a generalized knowledge of antioxidants and their benefits, as evidenced in numerous contemporary studies.

CHAPTER ONE

Theories of Disease

A Personal Note from Dr. Balch: I was so very fortunate to have the greatest father in the world. I idolized him. He was a great urological surgeon and I wanted to follow in his footsteps. There were many times I literally followed in his footsteps because I would go with him on his rounds at the hospital. He had a gentle and sensitive bedside manner, which I absorbed and later used in my practice. However, I learned that it takes more than a good bedside manner, or even being highly specialized in a field of medicine, to get people well. It takes the knowledge of *why* they are ill and the ability to address the cause, not merely the symptoms.

Hold it!!! Now don't let a word like "theory" turn you off. It's important for you to know about theories because it affects the way you choose to receive your health care today.

Theories are also important to know about because you are personally touched by them. Today's modern medicine is mostly based on what is termed the "germ theory." I practiced it, my father practiced it, and most physicians that take care of you today practice it. So, it's important that you know about this theory, but I feel that it's equally important for you to know and understand how medicine is changing and how those changes can affect you and your family.

There is also the theory concerning the "whole." This is the theory that changed my view and approach to healthcare because it was this theory that I have found has drastically improved the health of my patients.

This new alternative theory is revolutionizing modern medical thought and dramatically improving the health of people worldwide.

The Germ Theory

Most modern medicine is based on the germ theory of disease as proposed by Louis Pasteur (1822–1895). In this theory, the body is viewed as a sterile machine that will operate properly unless a foreign substance is introduced. Hence, it is thought that when specific microbes enter the body, they produce a specific disease. To return the patient to health, antibiotics and various chemicals are used to destroy these organisms. No microbes, no sickness. Health is defined as the absence of any germ that might cause disease.

This theory tends to view the body systemically: that is, some viruses affect the digestive tract, some bacteria infect the respiratory system, and the sickness is thought to reside in that system. Even the division of specialties in the medical profession show that illness is viewed systemically. Your gastroenterologist cannot help you with a sinus infection, and no urologist would dare to advise an asthma patient. The basic thought is that sickness is localized in one system and that health will be restored when the microbes are removed from that system. This assumes that the rest of the body is healthy and only this one part needs help. It also assumes that microbes are foreign to the body's natural state and function. The goal of medicine using this theory is to make sure that each body system works properly, and it will if it is free from bacterial and viral infection.

The famous French physiologist Claude Bernard (1813–1878) understood the concept of the whole. He emphasized the importance of the body's internal environment. In contrast to the prevalent doctrine of Pasteur, he taught that microbes (*e.g.*, bacteria, viruses) could not produce disease unless the "milieu" was unbalanced and conducive to the development of disease. His theory was that the whole must be sick before any germ can make us ill.

Renowned microbiologist René Debous agreed with this basic principle, saying, "[m]ost microbial diseases are caused by organisms *present* in the body of a normal individual. They become the cause of disease when a disturbance arises which upsets the equilibrium of the body." In other words, it is not the presence of bacteria or viruses that cause disease; it is the imbalance of the body's normal functions that fails to hold the microbes in check. The microbes are always there—in fact, some are absolutely necessary to the body's functions—but they only cause disease if the body is in a weakened or upset state.

Royal R. Rife, the genius microscopist of the 1930s, found that by altering the environment he could change harmless bacteria into deadly ones. More importantly, by returning the environment to a state of wholeness, the potentially deadly microbes could again be rendered harmless.

Yes, there are certain deadly organisms that even the healthiest body cannot overcome (*e.g.*, the TB bacteria and the cancer microbe); however, even in those cases, *the severity of the disease is always inversely proportional to the state of the body's internal environment and defense system* (*i.e.*, immunity).

A poorly balanced milieu results in reduced immunity and more serious disease. Degenerative disease—the kind involving the progressive deterioration of an organ or body system, such as cancer, diabetes, or Alzheimer's—results from instability of the internal environment and is only secondarily affected by the alien microbes. Degenerative disease results from an imbalance of the whole, a chaos and discord of the milieu. Interestingly, Pasteur denounced his own theory on his death bed: "Bernard is right. The microbe is nothing. The environment is all important."

The Wholeness Theory

"Being whole" is the key to better health. If the whole of the environment is disturbed from its healthy whole condition, disease is inevitable. This is not solely because of a foreign invader, but because of an imbalance and malnourished milieu: the "whole."

Wholeness might be defined as health restored. Here the internal environment of the body is stabilized and in perfect balance. This is balance at all levels, from the whole to each system, to each organ, to each cell, to each chemical reaction in the cells. It is particularly these smallest levels that affect us most, for when the cells do not work properly, the organ malfunctions. But many of the reasons for problems at the chemical level have to do with lifestyle choices that the whole person makes and lives out. All effective remedies for disease must take into consideration the whole person. Restoration of the body's health (wholeness), begins with an understanding that supplying the body with "good things" is foundational to becoming whole.

The wholeness theory can be broken down into three sub–areas: 1) Good Things for the Body, 2) Good Things for the Soul, and 3) Good Things for the Spirit.

Good Things for the Body

Wholeness must begin with providing the body with all that it needs to maintain its proper functioning. This means we must maintain a balance of activity and rest, of heat and cold, of fat and lean, for any extreme of these things leads to imbalance and sickness. Fatigue and hyperthermia stress the body so that we are much more likely to succumb to disease in these states. We must also have proper hydration and a good balance of the nutrients needed for the cellular activity we will describe in this book. For most of us, that means nutritional supplementation because our diets simply cannot give us all that we need.

Counterfeit foods, those created by man, are unable to supply what the body needs to maintain this stability and wholeness. Wholeness cannot be attained from them. Do not be deceived. Although today's foods look good and taste good, they are lacking in nutritional substance and often contain toxic substances that damage and destroy the internal environment. Now, God's food contains the life force—the essential nutrients, enzymes, et cetera—that are necessary to maintain the body's healing force within. Without them, the body perishes before its time.

Those foods that have been designed by God prevent disease and heal disease. Man's attempts to improve on God's foods have been a failure. Paradoxically, these counterfeit foods often cause the very diseases we confront everyday.

Good Things for the Soul

Along with the physical stresses we encounter, there are emotional stresses, too. These put just as much stress on the body as physical factors do, and often more! Notice that it is the *body* that takes the burden of *emotional* stress.

To maintain health, we must learn to nourish our soul and give it all that it needs to stay in balance. No one can live an emotionless life. Those who try are simply repressing their feelings, which magnifies emotional stress, and the body reacts by becoming ill with colitis, migraines, ulcers, cancer, and other maladies. But we can learn to balance negative emotions with positive ones. Here are some simple suggestions:

- Limit the time spent in worry. Set aside an hour or so each week for concentrated worry, then go enjoy your life the rest of the week.

- Cultivate friendships with people who can support and uplift you, and you can do the same for them.

- Music nourishes the soul. It allows for emotional response not directed at any particular problem in life and expands your connection to humanity.

- Get a massage. While this seems like a physical therapy, it does wonders for the emotions. It creates peace and releases emotional tension built up in the muscles.

- Laugh—out loud, long and hard. We are seeking balance. The worse you feel, the more you need a good laugh.

Good Things for the Spirit

The best definition of spirituality is: seeking to know where you fit in with everything. Man, being created in God's (Spirit) image, is a spirit, residing in his body, possessing his soul.

Balance is maintained by acknowledging that there is a power greater than us that has created us. Indeed, we are "fearfully and wonderfully made." Next, we must learn that we are not God. He is infinitely good, all-knowing, and all-powerful. We have some good, some knowledge, and some power, but we spend most of our lives dealing with the consequences of the harm we have caused ourselves and others out of ignorance and an inability to exercise self-control. If these things are true, then the next step is to ask for help. We cannot find truth by ourselves, nor can we act on it to correct our relationships. We need enlightenment and we need help to change. Until we are in this process of changing to conform to the truth, we are out of balance.

What does this have to do with health? When our minds are corrupted by falsehoods and we make choices based on false information, we begin deceiving ourselves, rationalizing our bad choices, and running further from the truth. This in turn corrupts our relationships with everyone around us, even leading us to self-destructive behaviors. We then must live with the consequences of all those choices in an atmosphere of emotional stress, guilt, and shame. That directly effects our emotional state, which leads to chemical changes in our brains and our bodies that result in physical sickness.

The way to spiritual health is no secret. It will require prayer, meditation, and time spent in study and in reflection. It will also require service to others, for we do not know who we are until we reach outside of ourselves and learn to give. But mostly it will require the willingness to take responsibility for our lives and change. We must be willing to think again about our lives, and think differently, so that we may change the course of our futures.

Attaining wholeness, and then maintaining it, is a life-long endeavor. There is never a quick fix: no simple remedy and no magic solution. We must become accountable and responsible for our bodies, for our souls, and for our spirits. This may require a change of heart and a new understanding about our bodies and the nutrients needed to sustain it.

The Whole Person

When God created humans, he also provided all the nutrients we needed to maintain a healthy body. He did not hide those nutrients from us, and he didn't package them separately and write a book to explain exactly how each one functions, either. He simply put an abundance of nutrients in the foods that we would eat. These were not processed, packaged, artificially ripened, genetically altered, or overcooked. They were simply whole foods that God gave people to eat, knowing that they were life-bearing foods, containing all that man needed. All we had to do was to eat these foods, in all of their diversity, with some regularity.

Health and its maintenance are not, and must not be, limited to the body. A principle direction in assisting my patients has been to teach them the importance of maintaining a state of nutritional health. However, I have discovered that each component (*i.e.*, body, soul, and spirit) interacts and directly affects the others. Therefore, all three parts must be dealt with or restored health will not be possible.

In this chapter, I want to identify and briefly discuss this medically alternative "wholeness" concept for you. "Good Things for the Body" (*i.e.*, antioxidants consisting of vitamins, minerals, herbs, amino acids, enzymes, bioflavonoids, carotenoids, and other supplements) are discussed throughout this text and itemized in greater detail in chapter 5. "Good Things for the Soul" and "Good Things for the Spirit" are again addressed in chapter 6.

The Free Radical Impact

History of Free Radicals

In 1954, the free radical theory of aging was first described by Dr. Denham Harman, who declared that a "single common process, modifiable by genetic and environmental factors, was responsible for aging and death of all living things." He identified this process saying, "Aging is caused by free radical reactions, which may be caused by the environment, from disease and intrinsic reactions within the aging process." Dr. Harman's conclusion, written more than forty years ago, sums up much of what we finally agree upon today:

> The free radical theory of aging is supported by studies on the origin of life and evolution, studies on the effect of ionized radiation on living things, the dietary manipulations of endogenous free radicals, the reasonable explanation that the free radical theory provides for aging, and finally the increasing number of studies which show that free radical reactions are involved in the pathogenesis of specific diseases.

Yet, Dr. Harman's work was largely ignored and rejected. Even as late as 1977, authorities in the chemical field were still not convinced that superoxide could "Act as a deleterious or cytotoxic species in living cells."[1]

The idea that dangerous free radicals were present in the human biological system was considered untenable by most biologists until 1969. They were convinced that disease must come from outside of man, not as a by-product of normal biological

functions. At that time, a copper-containing protein had been isolated from red blood cells that had no known function. It was
then discovered that this copper protein also contained zinc. It
was an enzyme uniting two superoxide molecules to form one
molecule of hydrogen peroxide and one molecule of oxygen. The
protein was renamed superoxide dismutase (SOD) because of its
ability to combine two molecules of superoxide.

Since the subunit for SOD was superoxide, a free radical, it
became apparent that at least one free radical is normally found
in biological systems. With this revelation, research in this area of
biology increased dramatically, opening a whole new avenue of
discovery. Other free radicals were subsequently discovered. Their
scavengers were soon discovered, also.

And importantly, the generation of these free radicals was
not only related to the normal utilization of oxygen, but also in
the disease-fighting potential of the white blood cells produced
for the express purpose of neutralizing invading microorganisms. It was eventually recognized that superoxide and the hydroxyl radical were instrumental as causative factors not only in
many degenerative diseases but in the aging process as well. So
we have finally arrived at the point Dr. Harman had established
in 1954.

Fingerprints of Free Radical Activity: The HLB Test: Having established
the significance of free radicals in human biology, their detection, by
seeing their "fingerprints," was to be of great value to the doctor. A simple
detection system is the HLB blood test. Briefly, this test reveals the activity of such reactive oxygen species as superoxide, hydrogen peroxide,
and the hydroxyl radical by changed patterns in coagulated blood. The
biochemistry of these changes may be explained scientifically and seen
clinically by comparing tests from normal samples and those from people
suffering from various degenerative disorders. One example is the changes
seen in progressively worsening cancer patients. The HLB test provides
not only an oxidative "fingerprint," but a detection system for monitoring the progress of therapy.

Introduction to the Oxygen Paradox

In keeping with "being whole" as a key to maintaining the best of
health, medical professionals are beginning to address alternative
theories. One exciting new discovery is the oxygen paradox and
how to make it work to your advantage. Once you understand

what it is, how it works, and how to counteract it, it will literally change your life and the lives of your loved ones.

Chapter 2 delves into the study of oxygen and how it is both beneficial and potentially toxic to our bodies. So, to learn how to break the code of this oxygen paradox, just turn the page.

Oxidology

Oxidology, the study of oxygen and how our body uses it, has uncovered a fascinating paradox. We all know that humans must have oxygen to survive; however, as our bodies use oxygen, it becomes both a blessing and a curse, because dangerous free radicals are formed. How can oxygen, so necessary for our survival, also be our enemy?

Aerobic Metabolism

Aero-what? Scientists love to put Greek words together. In this case, the words mean something like "air-living change." So, aerobic metabolism is the process by which our bodies change oxygen into energy. We breathe air in and our lungs take the oxygen out of it. Our blood (specifically the hemoglobin) picks up oxygen and carries it throughout our bodies to each cell. Every cell uses this oxygen to create the energy the cell needs to do its job. That's the reason all those exercise tapes make such a big deal about aerobic exercise—it's the kind that boosts your aerobic metabolism, and aerobic metabolism is what makes us go.

Oxygen Depletion: Oxygen is the source of our "life-energy," but there is a problem. We aren't getting enough of it. The oxygen-producing forests are being destroyed. Modern industrial technology is polluting the air, further depleting the Earth's oxygen supply. In the past few hundred years, the oxygen content of our atmosphere has decreased by almost 50 percent.

Most diseases will not thrive in an oxygen-rich environment. That has been proven in the case of cancer. If there is enough oxygen in the cells, cancer and other degenerative diseases cannot exist.

How, then, does this lack of oxygen affect us? It actually causes us to make more free radicals. Boosting oxygen enables our bodies to get rid of free radicals better, but as we keep on living with an oxygen shortage, our metabolism becomes more anaerobic—as if we weren't breathing at all. Instead of seeking energy from oxygen, our body tries to find other sources and ends up producing all kinds of toxins, all of which increase free radical damage.

Oxidative Damage to the Body

As our bodies turn oxygen into energy, there are by-products that are formed. When you burn wood it produces heat but it produces smoke as a by-product. When your body burns oxygen, it produces energy and by-products called reactive oxygen species, or ROS as we will call them throughout this book. These are the dangerous free radicals, the oxidants that cause oxidative damage to your cells. What makes these by-products toxic is their reactive nature.

If you remember your high school chemistry, you know that atoms are made of neutrons, protons, and electrons, and that electrons like to form bonds in pairs. In reactive oxygen species, there is an unpaired electron in the atom's outer orbit. That unpaired electron doesn't like being lonely, so it tries to steal an electron, or maybe a whole hydrogen atom, from something around it. Unfortunately, what is around it is your body. So it tears a little hole in your cell wall, or changes the chemistry of the mitochondria in the cell (the cell's energy source), or it rips a little piece of DNA out of the nucleus. It doesn't damage much, but it damages important things. When you multiply that little bit of damage by the millions of free radicals created in your body each second, your body might qualify as a disaster area. Literally, ROS makes your body "rust" or "rot."

That's where antioxidants come in. They clean up as many free radicals as they can before damage occurs. Where damage has already happened, they come in to correct the problem. Sometimes the antioxidant gives the ROS an electron to stabilize it. Other times the antioxidant neutralizes the free radical by combining with it to form a different stable compound. There are also antioxidant enzymes that just help the ROS to react with other chemicals to produce safe substances. If you have enough antioxidants (good guys), they win and you stay healthy. If you don't have enough of the right antioxidants, the "bad guy" free radicals (ROS) win and can cause any of a long list of diseases.

Now, this is not as strange as it sounds. You see it all the time. Have you ever cut up bananas or apples to put in a salad? What happens to them if you set them out in the air for a little while? They turn brown. That is oxidation: free radicals at work. They eat up the cell walls and release the cell fluids, then attack other cells and make a layer of brown mush on the surface of the fruit. How does a caterer avoid this so that the fruit still looks fresh after sitting out for hours? He dips it in lemon juice—vitamin C! He fights oxidative damage with an antioxidant.

Just what is an antioxidant? It can be confusing because we talk about vitamins, minerals, hormones, herbs, chemicals, enzymes, and several types of food, calling them all antioxidants. So what we really mean is that *an antioxidant is any substance that can help us fight the rust-rot syndrome caused by free radical damage.* Most antioxidants are nutrients derived from foods, but there are a few exceptions, like the hormones melatonin and DHEA, and some of the enzymes your body makes naturally. It really doesn't matter where the substance comes from as long as it gets rid of free radicals before they can eat us alive.

What Kind of Damage Can These "Bad Guy" Free Radicals Do?

Plenty! We know that most degenerative diseases are linked to free-radical damage. That means diseases like arthritis, cataracts, diabetes, or any disease where some part of your body is slowly falling apart. They can also attack your brain and central nervous system, causing disorders like Down's syndrome, multiple sclerosis, and Alzheimer's disease. ROS have been strongly linked to heart disease and all types of cancer. They also weaken our immune systems in various ways.

Dr. Richard A. Passwater is an internationally renowned author and antiaging researcher. He developed the concept of the "biological synergism of antioxidants" in antiaging. His theory has been proven to be true. Antioxidants, working together, are a key to your health and longevity.

Free radicals have a penchant for attacking certain parts of the cell. Damage to these specific areas creates its own set of problems.

- **The cell wall:** It is normally porous, allowing nutrients into the cell and letting waste products out. When attacked, it can either rupture and leak or become clogged. Either way, the cell dies prematurely.

- **DNA:** When free radicals are in the nucleus of the cell, they are apt to attack the genetic material that the cell uses to reproduce itself. Sometimes a free radical will simply attack a gene and mess up this information, which is encoded by subtle chemical bonds. Another type of damage is called cross-linking, in which the DNA is linked to a protein chain so that it cannot replicate at all. These are now seen as the leading mechanisms for cancer growth.

- **Blood and tissue lipids:** Through a process referred to as lipid peroxidation, fatty cells in the blood and tissues are attacked by hydrogen peroxide or peroxynitrate (both are ROS). An example is low-density (LDL) cholesterol which, when damaged by free radicals altered by your immune system, becomes a bloated, sticky blob that forms an obstructing plaque in the arterial wall. This hardening of the arteries (arteriosclerosis) is a leading cause of heart disease and stroke. Fats that have been peroxidized can also become rancid and toxic to your body.

- **Mitochondria:** The mitochondria are the powerhouses of the cell, where cellular energy is created. If their reactions are interrupted by free radicals, then the cell does not have energy to work. As cells with low energy accumulate, you eventually have a whole body that is low on energy, tired all the time, and having trouble fighting off disease.

- **Lysosomes:** The lysosomes are little packets of enzymes inside the cells. These enzymes are designed to eat through anything except the membrane that contains them. When their membrane is ruptured by ROS damage, those enzymes proceed to eat through that cell, and the one next to it, and the one after that—and they produce more free radicals as they go.

This is bad enough. But as time goes on, the damage keeps accumulating. As our immune system gets weaker, the damage even speeds up. Eventually ROS damage produces all of the disorders we associate with aging.

Oxidation and Aging

Free radicals and aging are strongly linked. More than eighty age-related diseases can be alleviated by antioxidants that neutralize oxidant particles. These diseases that we doctors still attribute to your age really have little to do with time, but are directly related to the accumulation of free radical damage in the cells of your body. Age is related to time only by the rate at which oxidative stress is taking its toll on your body. And more important to you, that rate of free radical damage can be changed. Antioxidants are available that will dramatically slow the aging of your body!

As antibiotics in the last fifty years of the twentieth century helped "cure" many infectious diseases, so antioxidants will effect a "cure" of many supposedly incurable diseases in the twenty-first century and slow the process of aging dramatically. This is good news, but few of us, and I include us doctors, have ever heard about this antioxidant revolution. As you will discover if you heed the advice given in this book, there are tremendous benefits to be gained by slowing the aging process, not the least of which are looking and feeling good. If you consider nothing else, consider how much money you and your loved ones will save in doctor and hospital bills.

Aging might be described as that life process in which the healthy cells in your body are slowly but continuously being reduced in number. Aging is not, as is commonly thought, the inevitable "wearing out" of your body parts, as if your body were a car that needed an overhaul. It is the accumulation of damage done to individual cells all over your body that results in the problems we associate with aging. As more and more cells are affected by oxidation, symptoms of aging may not be evident, but the body is losing healthy reserve cells needed to react in emergency situations. When a crisis comes, there is not enough backup strength for that organ or system to function normally. This, in turn, leads to an imbalance in the various organ systems that normally would work together in harmony. As your body's homeostasis (balanced condition) is disrupted, all systems begin to fail, falling like a house of cards in the wind. Disease and premature death become inevitable. But the scenario can be changed if we deal with oxidative stress before these problems arise.

So, you can see that we don't age one day at a time; we age one cell at a time. That is good news, because we cannot turn back the clock, but we can prevent free radical damage from continuing to ravage the cells of our bodies. In some instances, we can even reverse this cellular damage. As we continue our discussion, you will see that many degenerative diseases are simply complications of accumulative free radical (oxidative) damage. But we have a choice about how this will affect us. We can choose to fight back.

Glycation and Aging: To be fair, oxidation is not the only issue in aging. Another important factor in aging is the process of *glycation*. Glycation occurs when proteins react with excess sugar. The resultant damage to the proteins is just as detrimental as free radical damage. These sugar-damaged proteins are called advanced glycation end products, or AGEs, an appropriate acronym since they lead to premature aging. According to Dr. Anthony Cerami, author of *The Glycation Hypothesis of Aging*, "The formation rate of AGEs increases as the blood sugar level increases and with the length of time the level is raised." The average blood sugar levels tend to rise with increasing age, primarily because our tissues are less sensitive to insulin. So as time passes, our blood sugar level rises, which causes AGEs to form more rapidly. Elevated and/or widely fluctuating blood sugar promotes the damaging cross-linking of collagen and other important proteins that is seen in aging tissue. As this damage continues, it leads to joint problems, loss of energy and muscle strength, decline of mental powers, difficulties with weight control, and a host of other problems we associate with aging.

You can control glycation, too, just as you can control oxidation. The answer is simple, but you may not like it. Sugar is not good for you. Avoid it if at all possible. Never add it to your food. If you must satisfy your sweet tooth, use Stevia, a safe sweetener from the South American "sweet herb" plant. You can cook with it, too. Another way to control your sweet tooth is to satisfy the dietary need that makes you feel that you need something sweet. Chromium picolinate supplementation (200 mcg daily) has proven effective for this by helping the body metabolize fats, carbohydrates, and proteins. It can also give you increased energy and suppress appetite.

Gain Control Over Free Radical Damage

While the damage from oxidation cannot be minimized, the body does have its own means of dealing with the problem of oxidation. The first line of defense against free radicals is a system of enzymes produced by your body to neutralize free radicals. They are superoxide dismutase (SOD), catalase, and glutathione peroxidase. In addition, the body uses antioxidant vitamins, minerals, and substances found in food and herbs to counteract the damaging effect of ROS.

Vitamins A, C, and E are all excellent ROS scavengers. Other important antioxidant substances found in the diet include:

- proanthocyanidins, in grape seeds
- herbs like ginkgo biloba and garlic
- quercetin, found in zucchini, squash, and green tea
- lycopene from tomatoes
- the trace minerals selenium and germanium, and many other naturally occurring substances, some as yet unidentified.

We will learn about these and other antioxidants and how they work in chapter 5.

But how and why do ROS attack cells? And how does the antioxidant system work to counteract this attack? This is best answered by examining each of the toxic species individually.

The Paradox of Oxygen: Now that we know how the by-products of oxygen damage our bodies, we may question the value of exercise, especially aerobic exercise. We have all been told that increasing the oxygen levels in tissues is beneficial to the body and that exercise should consist of at least twenty minutes of elevated heart rate and deep, regular breathing. To explain the paradox of oxygen we must remember that it is not the oxygen that is toxic, but rather the by-products of the metabolism of oxygen, formed as the body utilizes the oxygen. Increasing oxygen levels in the body is good, but we have to help the body deal with the by-products of using all that oxygen. The oxygen paradox is solved by boosting the antioxidant level in the body to assist the immune system in providing natural scavengers of these free radicals.

Antioxidants fight these toxic free radicals by combining with them, scavenging and eliminating their ability to attack the cell. To support this antioxidant activity, we must have available specific minerals critical to the synthesis of antioxidant compounds. These minerals include copper, iron, magnesium, sulfur, selenium, manganese, and zinc. If these chemical elements are not available in adequate supply, the defense system is compromised and unable to handle the toxic overload. The more oxygen the body is metabolizing, the greater the need for these minerals.

Specific ROS and the Natural Biological Agents that Protect the Body from Their Adverse Effects

Superoxide (O_2-^*)

In the normal activity of the body's processing of molecular oxygen, the free radical superoxide is formed. Superoxide is nothing more than an oxygen molecule with an extra electron. It's that extra electron that makes it a free radical. Superoxide is the most common free radical we encounter. Normally, superoxide is rapidly scavenged by the superoxide dismutase (SOD). This enzyme works by catalyzing (speeding along) a reaction between two superoxide molecules and two hydrogen molecules. However, if detoxification is not rapid enough (due to the unavailability of sufficient SOD), the superoxide attempts to regain an electron from any available source. Cell membranes are a favorite target. So are the mitochondria and the chromosomes. So, not only do we have a "bad guy" that may prematurely kill the cell, it may also create a deviant cell which could produce cancer. SOD, the "good guy" here, requires the presence of copper, zinc, and magnesium for its production and proper functioning.

Hydrogen Peroxide (H_2O_2)

One of the by-products of scavenging the superoxide radicals is hydrogen peroxide. It is not as reactive as superoxide, but it is not friendly either. You are probably aware of how a 5 percent solution of this chemical reacts when you pour it on an open wound. Can you imagine having the full strength stuff trapped inside a cell?

Hydrogen Peroxide is generally destroyed by either the enzyme catalase or glutathione peroxidase. Catalase works in water and glutathione peroxidase works in fat. When they finish, the hydrogen peroxide has been converted to water and oxygen (H_2O and O_2).

Hydrogen peroxide has been linked to the awakening of the latent Epstein-Barr virus, which in turn has been linked to chronic fatigue syndrome and aging. More startling has been the discovery that hydrogen peroxide has the ability to damage the master DNA template (your very own genetic inheritance) that tells the cells how to duplicate themselves. As with superoxide, these mutations open the door to potential cancer-causing activities (carcinogenesis), Down's Syndrome,[2] and other genetic diseases. Liver cancer has been directly linked to hydrogen peroxide.

One of the problems that you will read a lot about in the pages that follow is lipid peroxidation. Hydrogen peroxide is the chief culprit in that crime, and it causes a plethora of diseases in one way or another.

Selenium and L-cysteine are important in the control of hydrogen peroxide and lipid peroxidation. Both are necessary for the formation and replenishment of glutathione, which is the ultimate scavenger of hydrogen peroxide in fats.

Hydroxyl Radical (HO*)

What happens when there is not enough glutathione or selenium for the antioxidant enzymes to do their job? If hydrogen peroxide is not completely converted to water, the hydroxyl radical, a very toxic free radical, is formed. This conversion of hydrogen peroxide to hydroxyl radicals happens when metals, such as free atoms of iron and mercury, are present. Hydroxyl radicals are also formed during exercise.

The hydroxyl radical is the most highly toxic of the free radicals. It is so dangerous because it is *extremely* reactive, usually lasting only thousandths of a second before it steals a hydrogen atom from whatever it touches first. So, it damages the cell as fast as it can spread. It may not seem like it could do much damage in so short a time, but the fact is that you don't have any part in any cell that can afford to give up a hydrogen atom. And it never happens just one molecule at a time, here and there—it happens in millions of molecules at once.

Research has shown that the enzyme methionine reductase has the ability to remove this free radical from our bodies. Another effective scavenger of hydroxyl radicals is injectable amygda-lin (vitamin B_{17}—laetrile). This amygdalin is an isolate of almonds, apricots, and plum and cherry pits. Additionally, the proanthocyanidins found in grape seed extract and pine bark ex-tract counteracts this dangerous hydroxyl radical.

Singlet Oxygen ($^1O_2$)

Did you know that oxygen exists in more than one form? Normal oxygen, O_2, is good for us, yet singlet oxygen, $^1O_2$, can be ex-tremely dangerous. O_2 can be a very stable molecule, but if it is exposed to radiation in the form of sunlight, the chemical bonds break and it becomes quite hazardous to your health.

Singlet oxygen is involved in diseases of the joints (arthritis), but most damaging are its effects on the human eye. It can dam-age the lens, causing cataracts, or the retina, causing macular de-generation. In both cases, it is the exposure of singlet oxygen to light which triggers the ROS damage.

Now, a number of substances have been found to quench sin-glet oxygen. These include the carotenoids, such as beta-carotene and lycopene. Lycopene is the most potent of all singlet oxygen quenchers. Additionally, the tocopherols (vitamin E), along with the amino acid histidine, can neutralize this free radical. Even cholesterol can act as a scavenger of singlet oxygen.

What Factors Contribute to Increased Production of Free Radicals?

The production of free radicals is 100 percent normal. It goes along with breathing. But there are things that cause us to make more free radicals than we normally would. Here is a short list:

Stress—emotional or physical stress makes you breathe less and burn energy more. Stress feeds on anaerobic metabo-lism, not oxygen.

Ozone in the air—a great way to produce superoxide.

Auto exhaust—you breathe carbon monoxide and hydrochlo-ric acid instead of oxygen.

Cigarette smoke—same idea.

Inflammations—your body's immune system creates free radicals as it fights germs.

Radiation—alters molecules in subtle ways, throwing off free radicals.

Sunlight—a form of radiation.

Impure water—between the impurities left in municipal water supplies and the chemicals used to cover them up, most water is toxic out of the tap. Beware: bottled water may come from the exact same source!

Processed foods—you can't get nutrients from man-made food, so your body shifts to anaerobic metabolism to try to get something out of it.

Toxic metals—they are in our soil, our water, our air, and they attract free radicals.

Industrial chemicals—in general, man-made chemicals are bad for you.

Drugs—even the "safe" ones the doctor prescribes for you change your ability to metabolize oxygen.

So now we have identified the "bad guys." There are other free radicals that can show up, but we've covered the big four. We also gave you some hints that the war is not lost. There is a way to deal with all oxidative damage: we just have to have the right "good guys" working for us. As long as we have enough antioxidants in our system—that is, if we have the capacity to handle a lot more ROS than we are creating—we can maintain not only health, but youth and vitality as well.

In the next chapter, you will learn about the factors that increase our oxidative stress and how to combat them.

| CHAPTER THREE

Enemies of Longevity

A number of enemies are present in your environment, both within and without, that increase your risk of premature aging. While serving in the U.S. Navy during the Viet Nam conflict, I learned from the Marines that you first must know your enemy and his tactics before you can determine the best way to combat his attack. This principle also holds true in your battle against the free radical scourge that plagues us in the modern world. The following are some of the enemies that result in increased free radical activity in your body. They are enemies to your longevity and to your health in general.

Biological

Aging

Well, it happens to everyone and it is inevitable, but we don't have to help it along. We want to expand our lives, enjoy life, and be healthy. It's not about chronology, its about good health and a happy, positive attitude. Yes, it is about peace of mind. Your mind has a lot to do with aging. Remember that you're as young as you feel! You must have a positive attitude and not let your age prevent you from doing things you enjoy. And, with good nutrition and supplementation, you can slow down the aging process. You no longer have to expect to live with stiff, aching joints; indigestion; insomnia; memory problems; heart disease; cataracts; or macular degeneration. Granted, as we age, our eyes aren't as sharp or our bodies as flexible as they used to be. Do you know that 85 percent of our population over sixty-five in industrialized nations is chronically ill? We readily accept this as the aging process and feel it's inevitable. Well, it's not! As we approach our "golden years" it is the time to make sure we have a healthy diet geared toward maximum nutrition filled with foods that supply high levels of vitamins A, C, and E; carotenes; and minerals. These are all powerful phytonutrients that have antioxidant qualities.

You can increase your life span by changing your habits or life-style. Oh, it takes work, but you can do it if you want to do it . . . just take it one step at a time.

1. First of all, attitude is the most important. The mind can make you sick or well. It's very powerful. You must think positively. Be happy. Don't worry! If your thoughts are consistently negative, your immune system will be weakened and you will get sick. Remember: your health's first line of defense is always an adequately functioning immune system.

2. Moderate, regular aerobic exercise (walking is good) is very important in order to oxygenate your body. With exercise, oxygen and nutrients are carried to the cells through the bloodstream. Remember that diseases cannot thrive in an oxygenated environment. So, a brisk daily walk does wonders. It helps strengthen the heart, improving your circulation. Walking helps with joint mobility and improves your overall strength and endurance. Stretching and walking help to move toxins and free radicals— the very things that cause aging—out of the body.

3. A healthy diet rich in nutrients and antioxidants is very important to help you maintain an optimum level of health. Many benefits occur as the result of a healthy diet: better memory, more energy, positive attitudes, a feeling of well-being. If you can keep your internal defense system in tip-top shape, you'll be able to ward off degenerative disease that shortens your life.

Here are some dietary guidelines to help you obtain antiaging benefits:

1. Eat fresh fruits, salads, and vegetables—especially the green leafy, yellow, and red ones—as often as possible. These live whole foods contain the life-bearing enzymes. Try to

eat them raw as often as possible. Their juices are also very healthy. It's good to eat locally grown food. However, you should be aware that the soils in some areas of the U.S. are deficient in minerals (*e.g.*, selenium) and vitamins, which are necessary for good health. Therefore, it's important to supplement your diet with a good multivitamin, multimineral complex. Fresh fruits and vegetables provide the most vitamins and minerals, plus fiber and enzymes in proper balance: phytonutrients, working together (synergistically) to enhance each other's healing qualities. Try to cultivate a taste for them.

2. Whole grains, seeds, nuts, and legumes are also necessary in a balanced diet. They provide fiber to keep your body's digestive tract regulated. These are better sources for your proteins than meat, yet still supply all of your amino acid requirements. Amino acids are the building blocks of proteins. If you do eat meat, eat less red meat and make sure it's lean. Fish and poultry are also excellent sources of protein.

3. Have a mixed diet of as many different foods as possible.

4. Eat small amounts of low-fat cheese, eggs, and dairy products.

5. To keep your digestive tract healthy, you must eat foods that contain friendly bacterial flora, the acidophilus lactobacilli. These can be found in foods such as yogurt, sauerkraut, kefir milk, and cheese. Without these friendly bacteria, assimilation of nutrients is impossible. Malnutrition, decreased immunity, and degenerative disease result.

6. Drink plenty of fresh, pure water. Distilled water or ultrafiltered (reverse osmosis) water is best.

7. Keep your body more alkaline by eating vegetables and fruits, especially drinking green drinks. You can find all kinds of green powders in health food stores. (See chapter 5 for more on green foods.)

8. Fats and oils derived from plant sources are best. Eliminate saturated fats from animal sources.

Remember that we need to supplement our diets to make it through these tough times in a polluted world. Good supplementation of vitamins, minerals, herbs, and enzymes will arm you in the battle against premature aging from oxidant stress. Chapter 5, "The Super Antioxidants," can help you develop your own health battle plan.

Drugs

Drugs are drugs, whether over-the-counter (OTC), prescribed, or recreational. They all act on the cellular chemistry of the body and their use often results in a deficiency of various nutrients they deactivate and destroy. There are many ways drugs destroy nutrients in our bodies: through urinary excretion, stool elimination, blocking their attachment to cells, blocking their absorption, binding to them, inactivating them, causing rapid usage of them, and actually destroying them. All drugs are potentially dangerous!

Remember: the more drugs you take and the longer you take them, the more likely you are to be nutritionally deficient. Important nutrients such as vitamins A, C, E, B_6, and folic acid, and the minerals magnesium, potassium, selenium, and zinc, all so important in antioxidant activity, are easily destroyed by drug usage. Then free radicals can run rampant. If you are taking or have taken any of the following drugs, you are probably deficient in important antioxidant nutrients.

Aspirin—Isn't it ironic that aspirin is used to protect against heart attack and stroke, yet it produces antioxidant deficiency that leads to heart attack or worse. I take antioxidants (i.e., vitamin C and garlic) instead. I suggest you do the same!

Antacids—Tagamet, Peptal, Novocimetine

Cholestyramines (cholesterol-lowering drugs)—Cholybar, Questran

Blood thinners—Coumadin. Tylenol interacts with Coumadin, resulting in bleeding. This is deadly stuff.

Broad-spectrum antibiotics—Ciprofloxin, Noroxin, and many others

Antihistamines—Sudafed, Actifed, Benedryl

Anticonvulsants—Dilantin

Urinary antibiotics—Macrodantin

Corticosteroids—the Cortisone Boys

This is just a partial list of the OTC and prescribed drugs that can cause an antioxidant deficiency in the body. In addition, regular use of OTC drugs such as laxatives, aspirin, and antihistamines may result in a major nutritional deficiency! Also, products containing mineral oils bind to fat-soluble vitamins A, D, E, and K and deplete them.

So, you see how important it is to eat nourishing foods and to take supplements to rebuild and strengthen your body. Instead of strengthening the body, drugs weaken it because they weaken your immune system, your first line of defense. Be cautious! Learn about the drugs you are taking. Never, never stop taking a medication without the supervision of your doctor, and never stop taking a medication cold turkey! Educate yourself, your physician, and your druggist. Take control of your health.

Inflammation

All inflammatory reactions involve the release of free radicals in the body, either through initiation or perpetration. Inflammation is the body's natural reaction to infection and/or injury. Normally, the white blood cells in the body release free radicals to kill invading bacteria and viruses, but when irritated tissues become red and swollen, they release additional free radicals and put the body into an overload mode. If there are not enough antioxidants to counteract the inflammation, the result is chronic inflammatory disease, continuously overloading our bodies with damaging free radicals. Arthritis is a good example of a common chronic inflammatory disease.

However, these inflammatory problems can be prevented through sound nutrition and antioxidant supplementation, especially vitamins A, C, and E. The best dietary approach is to eat foods that strengthen the joints and build up muscles and connective tissue. Conversely, an improper diet can also directly lead to inflammatory problems that can be exacerbated at any time and become both painful and limiting. Because acid pH in the body promotes inflammation, it's very important to limit the intake of meat, eggs, dairy products, and man-made processed food, which, when metabolized, raise the body's acid pH level.

Here are some simple nutritional tips to help counteract inflammation:

- Eat plenty of oily fish such as sardines and salmon.
- Include foods high in antioxidants in your diet. Vitamins A, C, and E all counteract inflammation.
- To get enough vitamin C, eat avocados, asparagus, and sunflower seeds, not just citrus fruits.
- Olive oil is high in vitamin E and can be used as a substitute for other, less healthy oils.
- Eat raw carrots and broccoli as well as apricots, yams, cantaloupe, and cabbage.
- Make sure you eat foods high in the antioxidant selenium, such as shellfish, whole grains, and brewer's yeast.

All of these foods are alive with enzymes, amino acids, fatty acids, and antioxidants. Especially important are:

Enzymes. These proteins, especially the proteases, help control inflammation. Enzymes taken for this purpose should be ingested between meals so they will be attracted to the inflamed area and not the digestive tract. Enzyme therapy aids in controlling inflammation by digesting and removing accumulated debris. The enzyme free radical scavenger superoxidant dismutase (SOD) is especially effective in reducing inflammation.

Zinc. This cofactor has antioxidant supportive qualities and is important both in healing tissue and inhibiting inflammation.

Stress

It's barely 9 A.M. and already it's turning into one of those days. The kids didn't want to get up for school and when you finally got them dressed, fed, and ready, the car battery was dead. Luckily, your neighbor had a set of jumper cables but, after dropping the kids off just as the tardy bell sounded, you found yourself in gridlock on what is laughingly known as the expressway.

After more than thirty minutes of snail's progress you pull into the parking lot at work. It's just started to rain and the only parking space you can find is a fifty-yard dash away from the entrance of your office building. Using your coat as an umbrella, you make a break for the door, and you would have arrived relatively dry if it hadn't been for the miniature raging river that blocked the way to your goal. Your shoes and socks soaked, you stand waiting for an elevator that takes its own sweet time in arriving. Then, when you finally make it to your desk, there's an e-mail saying your boss wants to see you right away. Taking a deep breath, you count to ten and tell yourself everything's going to be all right. But, it turns out to be a day filled with unwelcome surprises. As a final insult, you step squarely in a present left by the neighbor's dog just before you reach the safety and security of your own front door.

Everyone has those kinds of experiences; occasionally, we even have a name for them, "bad hair days." These are the times we feel stress most acutely. But, whether we realize it or not, even a day relatively free from crisis can leave its indelible imprint on the mind, body and spirit.

Stress is the quiet intruder. While the morning just described is an extreme example, often stress makes us uptight and we don't even realize it. It's a part of everyday life and it can affect us physically, emotionally, and spiritually. In today's busy, complex world, we're constantly faced with job pressures, disagreements, decisions that must be made, and never-ending financial pressure. Stress is inevitable!

Stress is also caused by environmental conditions, even something as common as when it is too hot or too cold. Trauma produces big-time bodily stress, as do illnesses and toxins. Our bodies have checks and balances to help us cope with daily stress, but oftentimes stresses are enhanced when we become overwhelmed with accumulated problems. So, you see, we are all affected by stress in varying degrees. Unresolved stress can shorten your life and kill you! It is extremely important that you maintain good health to combat stress because you will always experience some degree of stress.

Stress-induced illnesses are rampant in today's life-style. Stress puts pressure on all your body systems, especially the adrenal glands, resulting in adrenal burnout and a weakened immune system. Antioxidants are used to enhance the immune system and support your overworked glands and organs. They are there to combat free radicals. As you have discovered, free radicals ravage through cells in the weakest part of your system, producing severe damage and resulting in various degenerative diseases. Heart attack, high blood pressure, asthma, arthritis, and a host of other ailments are linked to your inability to cope.

The key to combating stress is two-fold. First, you need to maintain overall good nutrition to support your immune system. Second, this good nutrition should include more plant proteins for the amino acids, and more vitamin- and mineral-rich foods such as green foods (sprouts and dark green vegetables), soy, sea vegetables, legumes, whole grains, seeds, and nuts. Stress and nutrition are irrevocably linked. Excess stress generates a poor diet, which generates poor nutrition, which depletes antioxidant levels and weakens the immune system.

Perhaps the smartest health decision anyone can make is to fight stress through the use of supplemental antioxidants. Vitamins A, C, and E, with selenium and germanium, are excellent stress fighters. B-vitamins help calm your frazzled nerves. Adrenal support is necessary also. Vitamin B_5 (pantothenic acid) is important here. Your adrenals, which really take a beating from stress, can be strengthened with green drinks, sea vegetables, licorice, bee pollen, royal jelly, and ginseng. Many herbs have antioxidant properties that help combat free radical damage related to an immune system weakened by stress. Garlic and ginkgo biloba are examples. A detailed discussion of these wonder herbs follows in chapter 5. Other herbs have antioxidant-like qualities in that they have a major influence on the nervous system. Catnip, hops, valerian root, kava kava, and passion flower are just a few for you to consider.

Put simply, the best way to fight stress is to improve your diet. Eat more raw fruits and vegetables. Drink their juices for immediate vitamin, mineral, and enzyme uptake. Avoid processed foods, dairy products, alcohol, caffeine, and junk food.

Finally, another must in combating stress is as your kids might say, to just chill out. No matter which method you choose, you need to unwind often and get your mind uncluttered. You can do this through exercise, deep breathing, hobbies, and just plain laughing! Personally, I meditate on God's Word when the going gets rough and I feel overwhelmed by it all. Other methods to consider for stress reduction are yoga, meditation, relaxation techniques, life-style changes, and the hardest of all—just saying NO!

Be wary of prescription and tranquilizing drugs that are addictive and require increasingly larger doses to get the desired results. These drugs have side effects and whenever your intake of them increases so do the side effects. Use these drugs only if you *absolutely* must! Instead, use a stress-reduction diet following these guidelines.

- Eliminate stimulants such as caffeine and cola drinks.
- Eat serotonin-containing foods including bananas, pineapples, avocados, tomatoes, eggplant, and walnuts.
- Make sure your daily-diet includes complex carbohydrates. They are rich in tryptophan, which the body converts into serotonin, a natural mood-enhancing hormone with a tranquilizing effect. Turkey, bread, pasta, and grains contain an abundance of tryptopan.
- Breakfast is essential to "stress busting. Your first meal of the day should be comprised of whole grains, cereals, breads sweetened with honey and dried fruits or fruit juices.
- Become a grazer! But make sure your snacks contain an ample amount of complex carbohydrates.
- Use stress-reducing herbs in your cooking. Rosemary, lemon verbena, lemon balm, thyme, nutmeg, and basil are all excellent stress-reducing herbs.
- Drink herbal teas brewed from hops, passion flower, or valerian. Remember, herbs are compact powerful foods that contain vital antioxidants.

There are four major categories of stress that can occur in any combination at the same time. They are:

- *Chemical*—including, but not limited to, pesticides, insecticides, air pollution, water pollution, heavy metals such as mercury (tooth fillings), lead (paint, pipes), asbestos (insulation), and radioactive waste.
- *Emotional*—family disagreements, financial problems, job pressures, illness and death.
- *Physical*—trauma injuries, such as cuts and bums, broken bones etc.)
- *Infectious*—pneumonia, AIDS, lupus, candidiasis, and Epstein-Barr

All of these stresses can depress the immune system. It is up to us to cope and compensate by nutritionally supporting our overwhelmed immune systems. If the stress in our lives is not resolved the result is unnecessary cellular damage from the onslaught of unopposed free radicals.

Environmental

Air Pollution

Automobile Exhaust

If you make the daily commute to and from urban America, chances are you spend a good part of your drive time in heavy traffic. These traffic jams are a double whammy on the immune system because, in addition to their ability to send our stress levels skyrocketing, they leave us no choice but to breathe air filled with nitric oxides, ozone, and other poisons. In fact, lead pollution remains a serious environmental problem despite the world's switch to unleaded gasoline and the millions of dollars spent trying to control it.

Exhaust fumes are irritating to us all, but more than that, they cause sensitivity to allergens and increase production of cytokines, the allergens that cause allergic reactions. Overproduction of cytokines contributes to chronic inflammatory conditions, disorders of the immune system, atherosclerosis, and cancer. However, research has shown that antioxidants, especially vitamin E in combination with the omega-3 fatty acids, neutralize cytokines.[3]

Smoking

For many years cigarettes have been targeted by the American Heart Association as the number one enemy of health in the United States. The print and electronic media have covered the numerous class-action lawsuits against tobacco companies as headline news, and the Surgeon General's warning is printed on the side of every pack sold in this country, yet approximately 25 percent of the population smokes.

Smoking is a deadly practice, not just for the smoker but for anyone who happens to be close enough to breathe a cigarette's deadly fumes. Tobacco smoke contaminates indoor air with over four thousand known poisons, many of which are carcinogenic. Serum cotinine, a metabolite of nicotine, was studied in a large series of active and secondhand smokers, in the home and workplace. The number of smokers in the household and the hours exposed at work were significantly and independently associated with increased serum cotinine levels. Reason: the gas phase of cigarette smoke is abundant in free radicals, including toxic cadmium, nitric oxide, carbon monoxide, and aldehydes. Recent documentation in the *JAMA* has sadly revealed a sophisticated legal and public strategy to avoid liability for the disease induced by tobacco use. These documents also show that American tobacco companies have known of the carcinogenic and addictive qualities of cigarette smoke for at least thirty years.

The good news is that antioxidants help reduce the adverse effects of all these free radical toxins. Antioxidant levels in smokers have consistently been found to be below normal. However, antioxidant levels can improve within days after quitting smoking.

Smoking's link to cancer is no secret. The free radicals from cigarette smoke damage DNA, the genetic code system within your cells. Because of this damage, mutant cell forms develop that in time may produce cancer. A study of one hundred men reported in *Science News*, March 1996 revealed that the fifty smokers who received antioxidants had 50 percent less DNA damage to their white blood cells than the smoker control group, who received no antioxidants.

Additionally, in the area of DNA and reproduction, cigarette smoking adversely affects sperm density, motility, and the form of the vital head of the sperm. There is a dose/response relationship between spermatogenesis and smoking. The fact is that male infertility and birth defects in their offspring are linked to the father's smoking. During my early urology years, my interest turned to male infertility. I discovered that all efforts to effect reproduction would fail if the patient continued to smoke. This proves why! Cadmium, a toxic metal found in cigarette smoke, and nicotine have been implicated as the sperm's primary adversaries. The antioxidant vitamins C and E and Co-Q-10 are sperm protectors essential to the sperm's genetic integrity, preventing mutation that would lead to cancer and birth defects in the offspring.

What makes smoking even more dangerous is that it diminishes everything within the body that could help you fight its adverse effects. As just mentioned, it alters white blood cells and weakens the immune system. Smoking depresses levels of vitamins C and E in the blood. The vitally important serum carotenoids (*i.e.*, beta-carotene and lycopene) are also diminished in the smoker).

As to heart disease, cigarette smoking nearly instantly induces leukocyte adhesion to the vascular wall and formation of intravascular leukocyte-platelet aggregates, explains Dr. Hans-Anton Lehr. Heavy stuff you're saying? Well, simply put, smoking damages the interior of your circulatory system and sets you up for a blood clot (*i.e.*, heart attack and stroke). In the same study, Dr. Lehr discovered that vitamin C prevented this intravascular phenomenon. What this should reinforce is that smoking is dangerous business, but if you cannot break away from it, at least take vitamin C (2,000 to 4,000 mg/day).

Why can't you break this addiction? Cigarettes are laced with nicotine, a powerfully addictive drug that works on the brain. Once nicotine gets its hands on a person's brain it is as difficult an addiction to kick as heroin! As Dr. Leslie Iverson stated in the July 18, 1996, issue of *Nature,* 95 percent of smokers who stop smoking start again within twelve months, just like a heroin addict." It takes time and a dedicated effort to change the chemical pathways in the brain that enforce the desire to smoke.

If you smoke, try to stop or at least cut down. Less than ten cigarettes a day seems to be a critical number in reducing the risk of disease. In any case, take a potent antioxidant formula. The evidence is overwhelming that antioxidants could save your life and the lives of your family members, too!

Drink lots of fruit and vegetable juices and miso soup to counteract and clear the blood of nicotine acid. Include lots of vegetable proteins like beans, rice, legumes, and grains. Meat-eaters will be surprised to know that if you combine these foods properly, you will have the same amount of protein as a steak. Be sure to have magnesium-rich foods like green leafy vegetables, whole grains, sea vegetables, legumes, and shellfish. Eat lots of foods like carrots, celery, and citrus fruits. Avoid foods that are high in oxalic acid like chocolate, spinach, and rutabagas.

Some smoking facts:

1. If your parents smoke, you may have inherited the habit of smoking before you were born by absorbing nicotine through the womb.
2. Heartburn and ulcers are more prevalent in smokers.
3. Smoking causes arterial spasm, a big contributor to high blood pressure!

Here are some frightening statistics:

1. Each cigarette you smoke takes eight minutes off your life.
2. One pack a day takes one month off each year of your life.
3. Two packs a day takes twelve to fifteen years off your life.

However, depending upon when you quit, your life expectancy can increase from two to five years.

Chewing tobacco is also very dangerous. Men who chew have a high rate of cancer of the mouth and tongue. Women who are subjected to secondhand smoke have an increase in cervical, uterine, and lung cancers. Secondhand smoke is also very dangerous to the babe in the womb and to children.

Quitting is hard work, but smoking is an awful, addicting disease. You can quit. You can do it! Your life may depend on it.

Indoor Air Pollution: The term "air pollution" conjures up mental visions of smokestacks spewing clouds of poison over a helpless city, the midday sun all but obscured by the dirty, industrial haze. But, while the systematic poisoning of our water, food, and air are grabbing the headlines, indoor pollution has become a major health hazard, especially in the workplace.

In fact, many times we are better off outdoors than in the privacy of our own homes. Indoor air ranks fifth in the list of top environmental risks to health and, according to the Environmental Protection Agency, it can be up to 100 times more polluted than the air outside. This pollution has a number of sources including dust, office machines, cleaning supplies, and (although in recent years this situation has been largely remedied by the "nonsmoking" or "smoke free" office), cigarettes. Indoor air pollution can cause headaches, dizziness, and irritation of the eyes, nose, and throat. Over an extended period of time it can contribute to heart disease, cancer, asthma, and other chronic medical problems.

Ozone

Most of us who were born before and during the peak baby-boom years are lucky enough to have memories of pristine, blue skies and rainwater so pure you could drink it. Unfortunately, over the last thirty or so years, even we have become accustomed to the dirty haze that hangs like a vulture over all the world's major metropolitan areas.

Somehow, smog seems to be the perfect word to describe the dirty air the majority of the earth's population must inhale and exhale thousands of times every day. But, far more than just an assault on our sensibilities, smog is full of ozone and other dangerous free radicals, with more than 20 chemical compounds that promote oxidative reactions. Ozone is a chemical alteration of the one thing in the air we need most: oxygen. Ozone's chemical make up is O_3. This very unstable molecule is desperately seeking a way to become a stable O_2 molecule. When inhaled into the human body, it reacts with the first tissue it contacts in order to fulfill that need. In the process, it damages nasal and bronchial tissues and produces large quantities of the toxic free radical superoxide, which further damages respiratory tissues. Research presented in *Respiratory Medicine*[4] indicates that many reactions from ozone are initiated by free radicals, and antioxidants are extremely important in protection against ozone. Antioxidant defenses are vital in protecting the fluid of the lungs' lining against air pollutants like ozone. Some very important antioxidants to combat ozone are beta-carotene and selenium. If you live in a smoggy city, really double up on carotene- and selenium-rich foods. (See chapter 5, "Carotenoids" and "Minerals" sections.) Eat foods such as cantaloupe, yams, deep-water fish, cereal grains, and brewer's yeast.

Food Contamination

In the twentieth century science has introduced us to many wondrous technologies that make life easier, more interesting and, in the case of medicine and preventive health care, help us live better, and longer. But, as with everything in life, there is a flip side to the technological coin. With each new day planet Earth becomes increasingly more overpopulated and, in a race against time, scientists are feverishly searching for ways to feed an ever-expanding population which not only consumes more food, but takes up land that at one time was used for growing food. The scientists' dilemma is easy to see but almost impossible to solve. To survive we must grow more food on less land.

In this quest to alleviate world hunger, scientists have come up with a myriad of methods to speed up the growth and extend the shelf life of all types of foods, ranging from fruits and vegetables to grains and meats. Unfortunately, these modem marvels come with problematic byproducts that, if not confronted, will pose a unique set of health problems never before encountered in the world. The foremost of these dangers confronting us is the man-made contaminants that find their way into our bodies through the foods we eat.

Chemicals and waxes are used to prevent contamination and spoilage of food that has to be produced in great quantities, stored, and transported worldwide. They're also used to flavor food and enhance their appearance. In addition, food-processing procedures such as smoking, grilling, pickling, and irradiation may develop chemical contaminants.

Our modern world has brought to us many wondrous technologies; however, with these technologies come many problematic by-products. Let's begin with the produce and herbs we eat and the grasses and grains consumed by the animals we ultimately eat.

First of all, most crops are sprayed with herbicides and pesticides to control the weeds and the pests. These chemicals are absorbed into the air, the water, the soil, and the grazing areas of our farm animals. So, not only are we introducing chemicals into our systems from the produce we eat, but also through the consumption of meats, drinking water, and polluted air.

Produce suppliers and large supermarket chains are now being asked to reveal all the herbicides and pesticides used on their produce. Encourage this practice. Demand disclosure of chemical usage. You can have quality organically grown produce stocked in your local food stores, but you must insist upon it. Organically grown produce is safe, is more nutritious, and frankly tastes better.

An area of significant concern is with the meat and dairy products we consume. Did you know that 40 percent of all antibiotics produced in our country are fed to or injected into our animals?

This is done to prevent bacterial disease. The antibiotics are absorbed ultimately by our systems when we ingest the meat of these animals. No wonder we are developing many antibiotic-resistant organisms. Additionally, higher doses of more powerful antibiotics are required to control these resistant "bugs." This is a very serious thing! These antibiotics destroy the friendly bacteria (lactobacilli) of our intestinal tracts, paving the way for all kinds of problems, including yeast infections (candidiasis), the most common of which is chronic vaginal yeast infection and malabsorption of vital nutrients.

Pesticides: Whether we like to admit it or not, we put pesticides into our bodies everyday through the food we eat and the air we breathe. Is this a health hazard? Well, studies by the Environmental Protection Agency indicate that about seventy different pesticides now in common use cause, or are suspected of causing, various types of cancers.

Studies using both wild and laboratory animals show that exposure to certain pesticides can cause cancer, birth defects and problems with the digestive and system nervous system. In addition, the incidences of many types of diseases such as leukemia, non-Hodgkin's lymphoma, and cancer of the brain, stomach, and prostate are higher among farmers who regularly work with large amounts of pesticides. Some studies indicate that exposure to even low levels of pesticides for extended periods can cause significant health problems.

According to the National Academy of Sciences (NAS), because growing children eat more food (relative to their size) than full-grown adults, they are at an even greater risk from pesticides. This risk is compounded because children's bodies are still developing and are more susceptible to a wide variety of toxic substances. Early exposure to pesticides can contribute significantly to neurodevelopmental impairment, dysfunction of the immune system, and a greater risk of cancer.

It is also vital to know where the food you eat comes from. Even salmon, trout, striped bass, wild catfish, and bluefish can be dangerous if they were caught in polluted waters. Fish taken from the Great Lakes are particularly hazardous because of the waste and other pollution dumped into them by some of our largest cities.

But imported foods, including grain, meats, fruits, and vegetables are more likely than domestically produced foods to contain or be coated with hazardous residue. This is important to remember because almost half the fruits and vegetables eaten in the United States during the winter months are imported. Much of the imported fruits and vegetables come from Mexico, a country that has no agency responsible for monitoring pesticide use.

Still, the blame for these foods containing harmful pesticides reaching our dining tables does not lie exclusively with the exporting country. Every hour, of every day, of every year, the United States ships an average of twenty-seven tons of pesticides to other countries. On the other hand, only about one percent of the imported food coming into this country is routinely inspected by the FDA!

Mail Order Produce: To make sure that your fruits and vegetables are free of harmful or even illegal pesticides you can have organically grown produce delivered to your front door by using the book *Green Groceries: A Mail Order Guide to Organic Foods* by Jeanne Heifetz.

Further, growth and female hormones are given to cattle to promote their growth and to increase their milk production. These hormones are ultimately transferred to us through milk, meat, cheese, and other dairy products. Just imagine what it does to our bodies. Female hormones fed to cattle are thought to be responsible for cancer of the uterus and breast, painful menses, and premature development in girls. But males aren't immune to the consequences of this practice either. Female hormones have been shown to cause both premature aging and impotence in men. Wait, there's more!

Consider waxes. Yes, waxes. What about all of the fruits and vegetables that are waxed? This tactic is used to keep moisture in and extend shelf life. Presently, there are six types of wax that the Food and Drug Administration has given its approval for use on produce. Interestingly enough, they are the same waxes we use on automobiles, furniture, and floors. These waxes include palm oil derivatives, shellac, paraffin, and certain synthetic resins. Some of the foods that these waxes are applied to include: apples, cucumbers, peppers, eggplants, citrus fruits, melons, squashes, tomatoes, and turnips. It's my recommendation that you soak all of your produce in a nondetergent soap (found in health food stores) or peel them before eating them. This will remove these dangerous waxes.

A variety of chemicals is used to prevent contamination and spoilage of food that is produced in large quantities, then stored, and finally transported worldwide. Many chemicals are also used to flavor and enhance the appearance of food. Also, chemical contaminants may develop during certain methods of food processing, such as smoking, grilling, and pickling. And remember, many foods are irradiated today, causing additional changes in the food that may be dangerous to your health.

Food additives can be divided, basically, into two groups: those that are added intentionally and those that are added unintentionally. Food producers intentionally add dyes, cyclamates, artificial sweeteners, nitrates, and many other potentially dangerous substances. There are many studies that link these additives to cancer, attention deficit disorders, and immune deficiency syndromes. Unintentional additives are by-products of storage and preparation of foods. Contaminants include: aflatoxin (a fungus found commonly in peanuts) and other fungi; parasites; *E. coli* bacteria, which are present in meats that have not been processed properly; and the salmonella organism, which contaminates poultry, producing serious intestinal disorders when consumed.

Although food contamination and food additives account for a small percentage of the diseases that we see, this problem remains an additional stress factor that our bodies must deal with on a daily basis.

Pesticide Abuse: Many dangerous pesticides have been banned by the Environmental Protection Agency, but a survey conducted by the Research Triangle Institute for the EPA estimates that outlawed products including chlordane, silvex, heptachlor, and DDT are still being stored in as many as one million American homes.

Of the 2,674 respondents who took part in the National Home and Garden Pesticide Survey nationwide, 60 percent said that the only safety precautions they took when applying chemicals was to wash their hands afterward. A whopping 67 percent said they disposed of concentrated pesticides by putting them out for trash pick-up, and another 17 percent said they just poured the chemicals down the sink, in the toilet, or outside on the ground.

Cleaning Fruits and Vegetables: While no amount of washing or peeling can remove all contaminants from fruits and vegetables, it is still an effective way to remove dirt, germs, and pesticides from their surface. Putting a drop of mild dishwashing detergent in a pot of warm water will help, but be sure to rinse the produce thoroughly to wash off all soap residue. In addition use a vegetable scrub brush on potatoes, sweet potatoes, carrots and other fruits and vegetables that you plan to eat with their skins intact.

Tear off and throw away the outer leaves of cabbage and lettuce that cannot be scrubbed as vigorously as hard produce. Likewise, cut off the leaves and the top of celery stalks.

Vegetables such as cauliflower, spinach, and broccoli that do not have a smooth surface should be chopped then washed thoroughly.

Industrial Chemicals

Industrial chemical poisoning can occur whether or not you work with industrial chemicals. You'd be surprised how pervasive these toxins are in your everyday life. You may live near a chemical plant and inhale its by-products in the air or live near a landfill where chemicals have been dumped. Everyday cleaning supplies, if accidentally ingested, can cause acute chemical poisoning. Chemicals can be absorbed through the skin, inhaled, or ingested. Chemicals such as chlorine, disinfectants, heavy metals, herbicides, insecticides, petrochemicals, and solvents are becoming part of our everyday life. They enter our bodies and inhibit the functioning of our organs, glands, tissues, and cells!

Our best defense is to increase our antioxidant intake and be really kind to the liver and kidneys. These are the filtering agents of the body. Some helpful antioxidants include (see chapter 5 for complete details):

Milk thistle, Oregon grape, garlic, and green drinks—strengthen and protect the liver.

SOD—counteracts free radicals and protects the body from pollutants.

Grape seed extract—acts as a powerful powerful antibiotic.

Cysteine and L. Methionine—remove toxins.

Vitamin E—a powerful antioxidant, rebuilds the body.

Selenium—works with vitamins C and E to detoxify the body.

Radiation

It is popular today to laugh at the mid-1950s science fiction movie Godzilla in which a giant mutant-monster born from the fallout created by a nuclear explosion rises up from the Pacific Ocean to wreak havoc on Tokyo. But, while this movie takes its message to the point of camp, it does underline one frightening truth: the world is filled with free radical radiation, most of which is the result of modern technological advances.

In fact, you probably come into daily contact with some of the worst offenders and, like almost everybody else, don't think we can live without them. For instance, significant radiation emanates from your television for up to a distance of ten feet. The computer screens many of us spend our days working in front of emit significant amounts of radiation, as do the microwave ovens we use to warm our lunches. On cold winter nights we retreat under the warmth of our electric, blankets which, while they may keep us toasty warm, are also dosing us with (you guessed it) radiation.

We don't even want to think about those high-tension electrical wires strung across our neighborhoods. But, there is no ignoring documentation that shows a much higher incidence of cancer and other degenerative diseases, especially childhood leukemia, in areas near high-voltage electricity. It should make you, as it does me, skeptical of assurances from the so-called authorities who tell us, "All is well."

Even the medical profession is guilty of releasing radiation into the environment. Every time electromagnetic radiation is used in diagnostic medicine, whether it be a CAT scan, MRI, mammogram, or chest x-ray, vast amounts of potentially deadly free radicals are released into the atmosphere. And, in the irony of ironies, we use radiation to both treat and assess cancer while knowing beyond a shadow of a doubt that radiation causes cancer.

Exposure to radioactivity greatly increases the need for antioxidants to combat its effects. Many of the health problems associated with radiation can be prevented by taking antioxidants including vitamins A, C, E, carotenes, selenium, zinc, and folic acid. If you know you are going to be exposed to radiation, it is a good idea to take antioxidants just prior to or immediately after exposure. in fact, a diet consisting mainly of foods with a high antioxidant content should be the cornerstone of your everyday diet and health plan.

Sunlight

Each summer millions of Americans flock to the beach, many of them in search of the elusive perfect tan. In our society having skin the color of a South Pacific islander has long been seen as sexy and attractive and remains so today even after the discovery that exposure to too much sun is an invitation to skin cancer.

In 1985, scientists discovered a large, ever-expanding hole in the thin layer of ozone surrounding Earth. This ozone canopy is nature's way of protecting us against the harmful ultraviolet rays that diminish cellular immunity and increase our chances of getting infections of all kinds. But, unfortunately nature could not protect the ozone canopy from us. For decades we filled the air with chlorofluorocarbons from aerosol spray cans, refrigerants like Freon and other fluorinated hydrocarbons, and industrial-strength chemical waste that destroys the ozone layer. The U.S. Environmental Protection Agency estimates that a 40 percent depletion of the ozone layer by 2075 would result in 154 million additional cases of skin cancer and an additional 3.4 million deaths worldwide.

These are ominous statistics, but that is not the only problem. The sun is a direct cause of cataracts. Doubling the exposure of present UVB will increase the incidence of cataracts by 60 percent, and there are already 20 million cases worldwide, causing one half of the blindness in the world today. In addition, surgery for cataracts in the U.S. accounts for 12 percent of the entire Medicare budget. Few recognize the health and financial implications of this enemy: sunlight. But even more alarming, UVB diminishes cellular immunity and our protection against infections of all kinds.

What must we do to protect ourselves? Move underground? Remember that you need sunlight to activate vitamin D, which is needed for healthy bones and teeth, and for the protection it gives against cancer. You will have to walk a narrow road here: enough sun exposure, but not too much. Moderation is the key! Here are some suggestions:

1. Limit your exposure to short periods, preferably early in the day. Never get sunburned. This leads to skin cancer, especially melanoma, the most lethal of all cancers.

2. If you must be in the sun, protect your face, where most skin cancers occur, especially your nose. Wear a broad-brimmed hat that shades your face. Wearing the right clothing in the sun is important, too. Silk and cotton offer the best protection. Dark colors absorb the UVB more completely, so wear white or light-colored clothing.

3. Use a sunscreen. This is effective in preventing skin lesions that turn into cancer.

4. Take an antioxidant supplement. The following have all been shown to be protective of the skin and are immune system enhancers as well: the carotenoids; beta-carotene and lycopene; vitamins C and E; Lipoic acid; and Co-enzyme Q-10. Take a vitamin D_3 product if you are not able to get any sun.

Toxic Metals

Heavy metal pollution is plaguing America and threatening the health and lives of millions of people. Scientists are finding high levels of copper, lead, cobalt, mercury, aluminum, and cadmium in our soil and water. Also, items like cosmetics, cooking utensils, fabric softeners, some paints, plastics, polishes, solvents, and dental fillings can contain these dangerous metals.

What makes heavy metal intoxification so deadly is that it is accumulative. Once it gets into the body, it stays there. Various metals are attracted to different body parts and wreak havoc there, such as mercury to the central nervous system and aluminum to the brain. Lead contributes to lower intelligence in children. The presence of heavy metals in our tissues blocks the entrance of nutrients into the cells and the removal of wastes out of them. These metals destroy antioxidants, taking away our first line of defense.

People who are dentists, jewelers, painters, mechanics, road workers, artists, and dialysis patients are at risk of heavy metal toxicity. Lead can enter your environment quite easily. Residue of leaded gas is found in soil near roadways. It can be tracked into the house on the bottoms of your shoes. Cooking with bowls that have certain glazes on them may allow lead to leach into your food. And don't forget your water pipes. Some older homes have lead pipes or copper pipes that have been soldered with lead. This leaches into your drinking water. Leaded paint and little children is a very dangerous combination. Little ones put everything into their mouths!

Lead is far from the only culprit, however. Copper, another metal widely used in the United States, is in the plumbing of millions of homes and, like lead, it leaches into the drinking water. If you have fillings, you have mercury in your mouth and every time you chew, small particles are released into your body. Aluminum, the most widely used heavy metal, is a major factor in Alzheimer's disease and can enter the body in a variety of ways. Much of the cookware we use and the foil in which we wrap our food is aluminum, and the antacids we take and the deodorants we apply in the morning also contain aluminum.

Cadmium, which depletes and replaces the body's reserves of zinc in the liver and kidneys, is particularly dangerous because of the damage it inflicts on the immune system. Tobacco smoke, even second-hand smoke, contains cadmium and, believe it or not, it is present in grains, rice, coffee, tea, and soft drinks. Other common sources of cadmium are plastics, fertilizers, pesticides, soil, and the water we drink and the air we breathe.

Because of the proliferation of heavy metals in our bodies and in the environment, extra doses of antioxidants are crucial in order to counteract the effects of metal poisoning. Here are some important points to remember:

> Extra doses of antioxidants are crucial in order to block the effects of metal poisoning.
>
> Cysteine combines with copper in the blood and can help to pull it out of certain organs.
>
> Glutathione and L. Methionine help detoxify these metals.
>
> Selenium neutralizes the effects of toxic metals.
>
> Vitamin E works with selenium to neutralize toxic metals.
>
> Heavy doses of vitamin C help neutralize these particles and draw them out of the body.
>
> Garlic and apple pectin bind with toxic metals.
>
> Calcium prevents lead from being deposited in the body and prevents aluminum absorption.
>
> Zinc prevents cadmium levels from increasing.

Water

"Water, water everywhere, but not a drop to drink."

And I am not talking about the shipwrecked sailor. It's probably true in your locale, especially if you live in a large city. In 1988, the U.S. Department of Public Health warned that 85 percent of our water in the U.S. was contaminated to some degree. Water from some cities may contain as many as five hundred different disease-causing bacteria, viruses, and parasites. Unfortunately, this statistic has not improved in the last decade. Not only is our water contaminated, it is chlorinated, fluoridated, and in some cases, toxic ammonia had been added. Recently, the pathogen cryptosporidium has entered the water supply of several large cities, causing thousands of people to become ill.

There are other problems with our public water supply, too. Not only have water purification systems been known to break down, but pipes and solder leak poisonous lead into the water, lead that ultimately ends up in our bodies. We have discovered how poisonous lead and copper are to our systems.

In addition, chlorine reacts with organic materials to make carcinogenic substances, such as chloroform, and to further complicate matters, pesticides and industrial chemicals are contaminating our ground water. Most, if not all, of the great underground aquifer lakes are polluted. All these poisons are carcinogenic and cause free-radical formation in the body.

Poisoned Water: Most of us would like to think that the water that pours from our faucets is free of contaminants. But, in reality, an estimated 20 percent of the people in the United States are drinking water so impure that it violates safety standards set forth in the Clean Water Act.

In 1996, an estimated 90 percent of the country's public water facilities were still using contaminant-removing technologies developed before 1920. In fact, there is so much lead, radioactive material, feces, and other contaminants in our water supply that both the Centers for Disease Control in Atlanta and the Food and Drug Administration (FDA) urge people with weakened immune systems to drink only water that has been boiled or filtered.

Their advice is well given even for people without chronic health problems. According to scientists at the Massachusetts Institute of Technology, drinking water contains the microorganism *Helicobacter pylori*, which is suspected of causing stomach ulcers and cancer of the stomach. In addition, between 1986 and 1996 there have been six confirmed outbreaks of cryptosporidium infection affecting between 400,000 and 7 million people a year. In 1993, an outbreak of this single-cell parasite in Milwaukee caused an estimated 370,000 people to become ill and may have led to 142 deaths.

Despite this astounding figure, less than 10 percent of the 4.6 million home water-purification systems sold in this country in 1994 protected against cryptosporidium.

Next to oxygen, water is the most important element for sustaining life. We can live for a while without food, but only forty-eight hours without water. Water makes up 70 percent of our bodies' weight, with the average adult having about sixteen gallons of water in his or her system.

Water is so important for the functioning of our bodies. Water lubricates all of our moving parts and regulates all body processes such as digestion, elimination, circulation, and absorption. Water also transports nutrients through the body, dilutes toxins, and flushes out waste and poisons. Water is essential in controlling body temperature as well.

If we don't drink enough water daily, we'll become dehydrated. Signs of dehydration include: fatigue, frontal headaches, kidney disease, constipation, arthritis, circulatory diseases, and colds.

Remember, not all water is created equal! Eliminate tap water from your diet if possible. Chlorine and fluoride are poisons. Drink at least eight 8-ounce glasses of good, pure water per day. Get a good in-home water filter or drink bottled water. I have long preferred steam-distilled water. Distilled water is healthier for you, tastes better, and will not leach minerals from your bones and organs. I have recently been introduced to Oxy-Water™, which contains 34 mg of pure O_2 added to each liter of filtered and distilled water.

CHAPTER FOUR

Reactive Oxygen Species in Specific Diseases

This chapter will discuss several diseases that are generated by reactive oxygen species (ROS). Here you will find some facts about each disease, its connection with oxidation, and sources of super antioxidants to counteract it.

The terms "phytochemical" and "phytonutrient" may be new to you. *Phyto* is Greek for "plant," and familiarity with this term is important to your understanding of the foods I suggest that contain phytonutrients or chemicals! These are the plant elements that have antioxidant properties such as flavonoids, carotenoids, and enzymes.

Cancer

In the United States, a person dies from cancer every minute of every day. There are at least another 3 million to 4 million Americans who have cancer, and out of those, one out of three will eventually die from this disease. Although there are a number of varieties of cancer, there seems to be a commonality among them in that free radicals contribute in a major way to their development. And very important, antioxidants are effective in both the prevention and treatment of cancer.

Generally, cancers fall into four broad categories:

- Carcinomas, which affect the skin, mucous membranes, glands, and internal organs
- Leukemias, which are cancers of the blood-forming tissues
- Lymphomas, which affect the lymphatic system and are akin to leukemia
- Sarcomas, which affect the connective tissue, muscles, and bones

One of the driving forces behind my quest for better understanding health through nutrition was my inability as a surgeon to effectively treat cancer. As a urologist, cancers of the kidney, urinary bladder, and prostate were commonly seen in my patients. Although well trained in the radical surgical approaches to this disease, I soon discovered that cancer could not be cured with a knife, much as doctors before me had determined that tuberculosis could not be cured with a knife. The reason is that cancer is a systemic disease rather than a disease that starts in one organ and spreads. The problem is widespread to start with and must be dealt with in this frame of reference.

My exposure to a patient who had had his widespread prostatic cancer controlled and eradicated by nutritional support and supplements had a great impact on my medical approach some twenty years ago and forced me to rethink my position on the therapeutics of cancer.

Foundational in the disease of cancer is faulty immune function, and closely associated with this faulty immune function is the problem of reduced antioxidation. In fact, repeated studies have shown that the antioxidant levels in the cancer patient are dramatically reduced. A good example is in the prostate-cancer victim. Lycopene, a powerful antioxidant that prevents prostate cancer, is consistently low.

Of primary importance in the prevention and treatment of cancer is how the liver is functioning. It is thought by many scientists that nearly 90 percent of all cancers are due to the effects of environmental carcinogens (cancer-causing agents) such as those found in cigarette smoke, adulterated food, and polluted water and air. Along with the excess exposure to these carcinogens, deficiencies of the nutrients needed for proper detoxification through the liver and through adequate immune function lead to increased risk for cancer. Simply put, exposure to high levels of carcinogens associated with a poorly functioning liver and its detoxifying enzymes significantly increases our susceptibility to cancer.

Dr. Michael Murray, in his book *Encyclopedia of Natural Medicine* (revised second edition) states "the link between our detoxification system's effectiveness and our susceptibility to environmental toxins is exemplified in a study of chemical plant workers in Turin, Italy, who had an unusually high rate of bladder cancer. When the liver detoxification enzyme activity of all of the workers was tested, it was found that those with the poorest detoxification systems were the ones who developed bladder cancer." In other words, all were exposed to the same level of carcinogens, but those with poor liver function were the ones who developed the cancer.

The liver functions as a detoxifying organ in three basic ways. First, by filtering from the blood bacteria, endotoxins, and antigen-antibody complexes that have originated in the intestinal tract. "When working properly, the liver clears 99 percent of the bacteria and other toxins from the blood before they are allowed to reenter the general circulation."[5]

Second, the liver-detoxification process involves the formation, and ultimate secretion, of bile, which eventually enters the intestinal tract, is absorbed by fiber, and is finally excreted. Obviously, if our diet lacks fiber, these bile toxins may stay in the intestinal tract, be reabsorbed into the body, and end up causing intoxication again.

The liver's third role in the detoxification process involves a complicated enzymatic process that neutralizes toxins. This particular process is where the liver is able to neutralize the effects of chemicals, hormones, and other unwanted compounds. Again, quoting Dr. Michael Murray, "[a] significant side effect of all this metabolic activity is the production of free radicals as the toxins are transformed. In other words, with each toxin metabolized, a free radical is generated. Without adequate free radical defenses, every time the liver neutralizes a toxin, it is damaged by the free radicals produced."[6]

Murray goes on to describe glutathione (GSH) as "the most important antioxidant for neutralizing the free radicals produced."[7] Glutathione is composed of three amino acids: cysteine, glutamic acid, and glycine. Also of extreme importance in this liver detoxification process are the minerals zinc and copper, as well as magnesium, and the important antioxidant vitamin C.

NOTE: Glutathione taken orally is probably ineffective in raising tissue glutathione levels. However, vitamin C helps the body produce its own glutathione. Other compounds such as N-acetylcysteine (NAC), glycine, and methionine, along with vitamin C, encourage glutathione synthesis. Once again, vitamin C appears to offer greater benefit in raising glutathione levels. In conclusion, of all of these agents, only vitamin C and NAC elevate the tissue levels of glutathione. Glutathione-rich foods include:

- asparagus
- avocado
- broccoli
- Brussels spouts
- cabbage
- walnuts

One should also consider the special foods that are rich in those factors that help protect the liver from damage and improve its function. These include:

- garlic
- onions
- legumes
- eggs

All of these foods contain high amounts of sulfur. Sulfur is extremely important in overall liver protection, *i.e.*, via glutathione.

- water-soluble fiber found in oat bran, legumes, apples, and pears
- broccoli, brussels sprouts, and cabbage, the so-called "cabbage family vegetables"
- artichokes, beets, carrots, dandelion, and a number of other herbs, including milk thistle, turmeric, cinnamon, and licorice spices

Of course it is extremely important not to damage the liver through overindulgence in alcohol. Drink in moderation (two glasses of wine or beer or two ounces of hard liquor per day is considered moderation).

NOTE: Silymarin (milk thistle) is a special flavonoid compound, exerting special protective effects on the liver.

Silymarin prevents liver damage by acting as an antioxidant. It is much more potent than either vitamin E or C. Further, it enhances the detoxification process by preventing the depletion of glutathione.

Tomatoes: You may say tom-a-toe and I may say tom-ah-toe but one thing's for sure, unless you have an aggravating condition, it is not a good idea to call the whole thing off.

Tomatoes, which are in reality fruit and not vegetables, are an extremely valuable source of antioxidants, especially the carotenoids lycopene and beta-carotene. Low in sodium and high in vitamins C and E and the mineral potassium, tomatoes help lower the body's blood pressure and tendency toward fluid retention, protecting the cardiovascular system.

But, for certain people there is a downside to eating tomatoes. Because they are a member of the Solanaceae family and contain a bitter, crystalline alkaloid, tomatoes can cause an allergic reaction and may aggravate the pain of arthritis. People who experience recurrent mouth ulcers and/or eczema should cut down on their consumption of tomatoes.

As a urological surgeon for many years, I observed many men with prostrate cancer. Not a good disease! But it can be prevented; tomatoes and tomato-based produces (i.e., paste, sauce, etc.) have been shown to prevent prostate cancer. It would be wise, men, to increase your tomato intake.

Cardiovascular Disease

Nearly half of the deaths in this country are attributable to a single cause: cardiovascular disease. Heart attack and stroke are the first and third leading killers of our time. They are considered "silent killers" because often the first sign of a problem is a fatal incident. But the most dangerous sign of this disease, atherosclerosis, or hardening of the arteries, is entirely preventable. In fact, most of the risk factors that contribute to this modern plague are easily identified and totally within our control.

Your heart pumps about 100,000 times a day. If it had a continuous stream feeding into it, it would pump 5,000 gallons of blood through 60,000 miles of blood vessels each day! Over the average life span, a heart beats 2 to 3 billion times without us having to think about making it happen, or wondering how fast it should be. It is entirely self-regulating and automatic—until there is a problem, that is.

How does this disease work? There are many different mechanisms at play in the progress of cardiovascular disease, but the clearest warning sign and most common cause of complications is hardening of the arteries. That is something of a misnomer. Atherosclerosis is more like a coating of the arteries. The problem is that the inside of the arteries becomes clogged with a buildup of plaque containing cholesterol, fats, and junk. This restricts the amount of blood flowing through the vessel, raising blood pressure and eventually causing complete blockage of the artery. There is also a risk that some of that plaque could break loose and flow into the brain, causing a stroke, or into the heart's coronary system, short-circuiting the heart's rhythm regulatory system.

The first step in the process of hardening of the arteries is that the lining on the inside of arteries, called the endothelium, becomes damaged by oxidative stress. This has been observed over and over. In fact, you can put a healthy blood vessel in a dish of hydrogen peroxide, which produces oxidation damage, and watch the endothelium dissolve. This creates lesions, or little wounds, in which "stuff" can get caught in stuff like cholesterol.

That brings us to the second step. Low-density lipoproteins, also know as LDL cholesterol, have a tendency to be damaged by those same free radicals that oxidized the endothelium. When the endothelium is damaged, the immune system immediately sends out cells to control the damage. The result is a big, puffy, fat cell that just loves to cling to the inside of the artery rather than flow through it. It is known as a "foam cell." The high density lipoproteins (HDL) don't have the same problem and even help to clean up some of the mess that oxidized LDL can make. Normally, your body can even handle LDL just fine, but those foam cells and the damaged LDL get sticky and clog up everything.

The third step is simply allowing this process to continue, resulting in layers of plaque on the inside of the arteries. This reduces the blood vessels' ability to push the blood along. The heart creates most of the force moving the blood, but each blood vessel also has a slight pulsing movement of its own to help the blood along. If there is a layer of hard wax between the blood vessel and the blood, this pulsing doesn't do much good. It's like getting a massage with a four-inch-thick foam pad on your back. Eventually this vaso-motion stops altogether because the vessel is stiffened by the gunk inside it.

As the plaque builds up, the lumen of the artery gets smaller and smaller, so less and less blood flows through it. Now, what happens when you put your thumb partially over the end of a water hose? You get less water flowing through, but at a high enough pressure to peel the bugs right off your windshield. The same thing happens when your arteries are restricted: you don't have as much blood flowing through, but your blood pressure goes sky high. The net result on your heart is that it has to beat faster to move the same amount of blood that it used to, and it has to work harder in each beat because it is facing more resistance. The sad part is that you probably won't have a clue that it is happening until an artery is 90 percent blocked!

What happens from there? If symptoms are identified before a major incident, a change in diet and lifestyle can do wonders to reverse the damage. If not, there are surgical procedures to clear out some of the blockage, but all surgery carries risk. The worst cases are those who never even knew there was a problem until it was too late.

Blood Pressure: It's called the "Silent Killer" and day-in and day-out it quietly, anonymously in many cases, goes about its deadly business. Hypertension, or high blood pressure as it is commonly called, affects more than 50 million people in the United States alone. Left undetected and/or untreated it silently destroys the body's internal organs and can lead to stroke or heart attack.

But, the body has a secret weapon in the battle against high blood pressure, the coenzyme Q10 (Co-Q-10), which can help reduce hypertension. In his book *Heart Disease and High Blood Pressure,* Michael Murray, N.D., points out that a deficiency of this energy-creating enzyme exists in 39 percent of all patients with high blood pressure. Although Murray admits that how Q10 lowers blood pressure is a mystery, he believes that the key is Q10's beneficial effects on blood cholesterol levels and its ability to stabilize vascular membranes through its antioxidant qualities.

At any rate, several studies have confirmed what many doctors fear: most Americans are not addressing their hypertension problems by changing their diet. As a result, doctors end up treating patients for heart problems, kidney disease, and strokes, all of which are preceded by and related to high blood pressure. But, fighting hypertension is not an impossible task. You can lower your risk of high blood pressure by making a few changes in your daily habits.

- Keep your weight down; extra weight causes the heart to work harder. The result is an increase in blood pressure.
- Don't smoke.
- Avoid overindulgence of alcohol.
- As a general rule, vegetarians have fewer blood pressure and heart problems than meat-eaters. Eat more low-fat foods including fruits and vegetables, whole grains, and nonfat dairy products.
- Get plenty of exercise, at least four hours a week. This can be easily accomplished by making a morning or an evening walk part of your daily routine.

- Reduce stress by practicing meditation.
- Don't automatically salt your food, and keep your daily consumption of salt down to 2.4 grams (about one teaspoon) per day. Use potassium "salt" substitute. Try "sea salt" or kelp.

Risk Factors

Smoking

There are several risk factors that increase the chances of a person's developing cardiovascular disease. Number one on the list is smoking. Smokers are five times more likely to have heart disease than nonsmokers are. The risk for nonsmokers who live with smokers is almost the same. There are thousands of chemicals in smoke that contribute to heart disease. They are transferred straight from the lungs to the bloodstream, where they cause oxidative damage to the endothelium and the LDL cholesterol, generating atherosclerosis. Smokers are advised first to quit and second to take at least one gram of vitamin C and 400 I.U. of vitamin E every day. The same goes for those regularly exposed to secondhand smoke on the bus, at work, or at home.

Physical Inactivity

Another key risk factor is physical inactivity. As a nation, we have replaced physical activity with emotional stress. Rather than working really hard, we go to work and worry really hard while sitting at our computer terminals, then we come home exhausted and fall asleep in front of the television. Our greatest physical exertion of the day may be pushing our office chair around our cubicle while remaining seated. Again, this factor is 100 percent controllable. Not only that, exercise would be the best thing we could do to relieve the emotional stress generated at work.

So why aren't we doing something about it? First, we think it is too hard. We just can't see ourselves in Claudia Schiffer's next workout video, jumping around in spandex with big smiles on our faces. That's okay. The good news for those who don't do spandex is that you don't have to. A twenty-minute walk around the block three or four times a week can take you out of the high-risk group. Studies have shown that in most respects, walking is just as effective as running to promote general health. It is even superior in that it doesn't put extra stress on the joints and risk overexertion. In fact, "hyper-exercise" produces damaging excess free radicals. No expensive equipment is needed, no memberships, no embarrassing outfits, no pumping iron or bulking up. All it takes is a little discipline.

The second obstacle we face is time. Isn't it funny how we will complain about not having enough time to exercise, but we still manage to watch all our favorite shows and see all the big movies that come out? We always have time for what we think is really important. Do we really believe that watching *Seinfeld* re-runs is more important than living an extra ten years?

The third obstacle is that we often work out for the sake of working out, and forget to have fun. Choose an exercise that you like. The best exercise is the one that you will do. If you enjoy swimming, do that. Consider water aerobics. If you enjoy basketball, put a hoop on your garage and go for it. If you like to bowl, too bad; bowling doesn't count. We are going for activities here that involve at least twenty minutes of movement, not two hours of standing around broken up by two minutes of exertion. Sorry, that shoots down softball, too. Do a little of everything. Have fun. Just remember that sitting around can kill you. It is really a matter of making a decision and sticking to it for a month. After that, it will become habit, and good habits are rewarded.

Type A Personality

One of the risk factors that we heard a lot about in the '70s is the Type A personality. This is the person who is an overachiever, a perfectionist who works sixty hours a week, is very assertive, and doesn't understand why everyone else isn't like him. Even though he rarely shows much emotion, he may be prone to outbursts of anger. This is the person who has set himself up to live in that emotional stress we have been talking about because he believes that his work is what gives him value. He is driven to succeed because, if he doesn't, he feels worthless. This is a lot of pressure to put yourself under. And emotional stress doesn't happen in the mind alone; that pressure comes out in your body. In this case, that pressure puts stress on the heart and raises the blood pressure. Rather than cholesterol blocking the blood vessels (which may also be happening), the person's own emotional tension restricts the movement of blood from the heart and through the arteries. Since the Type A folks are in the habit of not paying attention to their bodies or their emotions, they can literally work themselves to death.

"But that is my *personality*. That's just the way I am. I can't change that." *Au contraire, mon frère.* If people cannot change, we have no business trying to rehabilitate criminals, and every church, AA group, psychologist, and school in the country should shut down right now. The fact is that we change all the time, sometimes depending on the group of people we are with. Change is the one constant in life. You can either choose to change in a particular direction, or you can just go with the flow and let everything outside yourself define who you are.

Sometimes we confuse personality with personhood. Personhood we can't change; it has to do with what we are. By nature, we possess the attributes of personhood. We think, we feel, we choose. That is part of being human. Personality is the sum total of what we have thought, felt, and chosen about everything that has happened to us up to this moment in our lives. Personhood is what we are; personality is what we become. It is how we have expressed our personhood, and it changes constantly. While we can't change our past experience, we can reframe it and choose to think and feel differently about it. We can also dilute it by putting in new messages, so that the past is not as important as it was when that was all we had. We can even expand on the past by learning new and different things, broadening our perspective. Always, we have a choice about how we have responded to what is in our minds, and we can choose to be different. It is personhood that gives us value: the fact that we have the ability to choose who we become. Personality is simply the net result of our personhood.

Long story short: You can choose to not be Type A anymore. You can learn to leave the office at five o'clock. You can learn to be less critical of yourself. You can even learn to accept things beyond your control. It is a matter of choice, and your heart will thank you for lightening up.

There are plenty of things we can do nutritionally to reduce our risks also. The most important of these relate to our fat intake and our antioxidant consumption. In addition to these, low levels of magnesium and potassium are related to increased heart disease. Diabetics are at increased risk of cardiovascular disease, about three times more risk, because of their impaired ability to metabolize sugars and fats. Platelet aggregation, fibrogen formation, and elevated homocysteine are blood abnormalities associated with heart disease that can also be controlled by diet.

Elevated Cholesterol

Cholesterol is made of protein molecules that carry fat (in the form of triglycerides) in the blood. There are four types of cholesterol: VLDL (very low-density lipoproteins), LDL (low-density lipoproteins), HDL (high-density lipoproteins), and the very dangerous lipoprotein A, which has a structure like LDL but with an adhesive protein around it called apolipoprotein "A." These are the damaged LDL molecules we talked about earlier.

Now, let's simplify that. Too much LDL and VLDL are both bad. LpA is contaminated LDL. So we can lump all three of those together as the bad guys, and HDL is the only good guy. Both low and high density lipoproteins do important jobs, but it is LDL that can be affected by oxidative damage to form the foam cells that are killers.

The job of LDL is to transport fats from the liver to body cells. HDL takes fats back to the liver. The total amount of cholesterol of all kinds in the blood should be about 200 mg/dl. LDL should be lower than 130 mg/dl and HDL should be higher than 35 mg/dl. The total amount of triglycerides they are carrying should be less than 150 mg/dl. If your LDL is too high, it means an increased risk of heart attack and stroke. The goal is to raise your HDL and lower the LDL.

How do you do that? The quickest way to change the kind of fat in your bloodstream is to change the kind of fat you eat. That is the reason people keep talking about saturated fats, polyunsaturated fats, and monounsaturated fats. Saturated fats raise LDL cholesterol, period! Saturated fats are easy to recognize when they are all by themselves: they remain solid at room temperature. Shortening and margarine are the worst. That strip of white stuff around your T-bone steak is totally saturated, too. Most of the time saturated fats are mixed with unsaturated fats and hidden, so you have to read labels. The best kinds of oils to cook with are canola oil, which is the oil highest in monounsaturated fat, and olive oil, which runs a close second but adds flavor and other benefits. Just by cooking with these oils, avoiding shortening and margarine, and limiting the total amount of fat you eat, your blood profile will change.

Another way is to eat oils that actually lower LDL and triglycerides. These oils are known as Omega 3 fish oils, or essential fatty acids. These oils come from cold-water fish like salmon, mackerel, herring, and halibut. The highest degree of heart disease is found in people with the lowest levels of Omega 3 oils. Conversely, you don't hear much about heart disease in Japan because half of their diet is sushi and the other half is steamed vegetables. Omega 3 oils will actually lower blood levels of LDL and triglycerides, reduce platelet aggregation, and lower blood pressure. You can get Omega 3s either by eating these fish at least twice a week, or by taking a supplement in capsule form. (Tip: If you take the capsules, you may find that the fish oil will repeat on you. Chewing a lecithin tablet when you take the capsule will solve that problem.)

Blood Chemistry Abnormalities

There are also risk factors relating to blood chemistry that can be controlled through nutrition. Platelets are the cells that are responsible for making the blood clot. Normally, they are spread evenly throughout your blood, but if they start clumping together, they form a soft clot traveling through your bloodstream. If the clot doesn't break up when it hits a smaller vessel it can block the vessel. This is especially dangerous in the brain. We call this problem platelet aggregation. The solution is to keep your cholesterol profile under control with Omega 3s and keep your antioxidant levels up. One antioxidant that is especially helpful in this regard is garlic, especially aged garlic (Kyolic). Vitamin B_6 (pyridoxine) also inhibits platelet aggregation and lowers total plasma cholesterol.

A second blood abnormality associated with increased risk of cardiovascular disease is fibrogen formation. Fibrogen is also an important protein involved in the clotting process, but if it forms when it is not supposed to, it makes the blood thick and stimulates the formation of plaque. Again, exercise, garlic, Omega 3 oils, and vitamin B_3 (niacin) can eliminate this risk factor.

The third irregularity of the blood is elevated homocysteine.

Homocysteine is an amino acid in the process of changing from methionine to cysteine (one amino acid to another). Normally, it makes the conversion to cysteine and blood levels remain stable, but if it gets stuck in this transitional phase, homocysteine begins to accumulate in the blood. Usually that happens in people who don't get enough folic acid, vitamin B_6 (pyridoxine), and vitamin B_{12}, which are needed to complete the conversion to cysteine. Too much homocysteine directly damages the artery and its endothelium. Abnormal homocysteine levels are found in about 40 percent of all patients with heart disease. The solution is to take 400 micrograms of folic acid, 100 milligrams of B_6, and 1,000 micrograms of B_{12} each day.

Low Antioxidant Levels

Low antioxidant levels have consistently been associated with increased risk of cardiovascular disease. As we have said, it is oxidative damage to the blood-vessel walls along with LDL cholesterol that are the primary cause of atherosclerosis. These are fatty tissues and cells that are susceptible to lipid peroxidation, so a wide range of antioxidants is called for, the most important being vitamins E and C, selenium, and the carotenoids beta-carotene and lycopene.

Vitamin E may be the single most important antioxidant for heart health. It is readily incorporated into the LDL cholesterol molecule and protects it from free-radical damage. It also reduces overall LDL cholesterol levels, raises HDL levels, inhibits platelet aggregation, and breaks down excess fibrogen. While small amounts of vitamin E are protective, doses of greater than 400 I.U. per day are needed to significantly affect an existing problem.

"Smooth muscle cells" are another problem known to contribute to cardiovascular disease. This refers to abnormal muscle cells in the arterial wall and the activity of the enzyme Protein Kinase C. PKC plays a key role in the formation of these abnormal cells. Vitamin E (natural d-alpha-tocopherol, but not synthetic d-l alpha-tocopherol) has been shown in rats, rabbits, and humans to block the action of PKC and prevent the formation of these abnormal smooth muscle cells.

Vitamin E levels may be a better predictor of heart attack than cholesterol levels. Low vitamin E levels almost always precede heart problems. Ninety thousand nurses were given 100 I.U. of vitamin E for two years and had a 50 percent reduction in heart disease. Similarly, forty thousand male health professionals experienced a 40 percent reduction in their incidence of cardio-vascular problems when given a moderate dose of vitamin E.

Vitamin C remains the body's most basic antioxidant because of its versatility. It not only acts as an antioxidant, it helps the antioxidant enzymes to do their jobs and it regenerates vitamin E as well. That increases the overall antioxidant abilities of your body and allows you to consume less vitamin E. It also lowers cholesterol levels and blood pressure while promoting more of the good HDL cholesterol, inhibiting platelet aggregation, and strengthening blood vessels. It also blocks free radicals in the blood before they can attack LDL molecules.

Carotenoids have only recently been considered important to heart health, but the results are encouraging. A group of twenty-two smokers and nonsmokers were observed and encouraged to eat foods rich in carotenoids: carrots for beta-carotene, tomatoes for lycopene, and French beans, cabbage, and spinach for lutein. This added about 30 milligrams of carotenoids to their diet. After only two weeks, blood levels of carotenoids were 23 percent higher in smokers and 11 percent higher in nonsmokers. Smokers are gener-ally deficient in carotenoids, so this was significant. It all translated into 14 percent greater resistance to LDL oxidation in the smokers and a 28 percent increase in nonsmokers. That gives us one more weapon in fighting the plaque that causes atherosclerosis.[8]

Proanthocyanidins may be equally important in reducing our risk of heart attack. These very potent antioxidants are found in a wide variety of foods, but are extracted from maritime pine bark and grape seeds for commercial preparations. They are consid-ered to be twenty to fifty times more powerful than vitamins C or E in neutralizing free radicals. Being water soluble, proantho-cyanidins complement the work of vitamin C and have been proven to protect the lining of the artery walls, lower serum cholesterol levels, and shrink the size of cholesterol deposits on the artery walls. A normal dosage would be 50 to 100 milligrams a day, but for therapeutic purposes, that should be increased to 200 to 300 milligrams a day.

Many doctors, even cardiologists, today recommend the use of aspirin as a preventive measure against heart attack. They point to evidence that aspirin has "blood thinning characteristics" that reduce the risk of a coronary event and doses of 300 to 900 milligrams per day are often suggested. However, at these doses, there is also a very high risk of developing a bleeding peptic ulcer. That hardly seems like a reasonable trade-off, especially when there are better solutions available. Natural alternatives like vitamin C, Omega 3 fatty acids, vitamin E, and the B vitamins mentioned above all help to keep the blood healthy and avoid platelet aggregation. Garlic is particularly helpful in "thinning" the blood. In addition to all of these, I personally like ginkgo biloba extract because I know this helps cerebral vascular circulation and also microcirculation elsewhere in the body. Rather than working on the blood, it works to relax the blood vessels and open the flow of blood.

Every aspect of this silent killer is within our ability to control. Yes, it will require some changes in your lifestyle, but what good is your lifestyle if it costs you your life? I'd say it is worth the effort.

Vegetables vs. Meat: You don't have to be a committed vegetarian to have a healthy diet but, as an ever-growing mountain of scientific evidence shows, you are much better off when you make that steak or hamburger the exception rather than the rule. A diet rich in fruits and vegetables plays a role in reducing all the major health causes of death. However, while the evidence is overwhelming that a largely vegetarian diet is much better for you than a diet loaded with animal fats, it doesn't mean you should preclude meat from your diet entirely. Still, while meat does nothing to protect the body while doing at least a certain amount of damage, fruits and vegetables are your unflinching ally in the body's war against disease. Here are four good reasons, some directly attributable to red meat, for maintaining a diet rich in fruits and vegetables.

- *Heart Disease*—For two decades scientists have touted a high vegetable and fruit diet because of its low content of cholesterol and saturated fat. But, subsequent research shows that the soluble fiber in barley, oats, peas, and beans actively works to help lower cholesterol.
- *Cancer*—If you absolutely can't stop playing Russian roulette with cigarettes, at least hedge your bets by eating plenty of fruits and vegetables. Not only does this dynamic duo reduce the risk of lung cancer, it protects against many other types of cancers, including cancer of the stomach, mouth, prostate, gastrointestinal system, and colon. In fact, in a study of 50,000 men conducted by Harvard Medical School, it was determined that men who eat red meat five times a week are four times more likely to contract colon cancer as

men who eat red meat once a month. In the same study, the heavy meat-eaters were twice as likely to get prostate cancer as men who did not eat red meat on a regular basis.

• *Water and Air Pollution*—Believe it or not, meat does play an indirect role in polluting our environment. In addition to the chemicals, pesticides, and other poisons that get dumped into our drinking water and released into our breathing air, sewage from stockyards, chicken factories, and other animal facilities find their way into the water. Furthermore, an estimated 30 million tons of methane gas, one of the principal causes of global warming, is in our atmosphere because of animal manure and sewage ponds.

• *Safe Foods*—There's no doubt about it: eating meat is a riskier proposition than sitting down to a meal of healthful fruits and vegetables. In fact, some of the deadliest diseases on earth make their way into the human body via our consumption of animals. Ground beef, perhaps the most commonly eaten form of meat in the United States, is the most likely sources of *E. coli* bacteria. In addition, improperly prepared poultry is a breeding ground for Salmonella and Campylobacter. These bacteria that are pathogenic to human beings and animals can be present in raw vegetables and fruits, but they are much more likely to be found in poultry. Even seafood, if tainted or improperly prepared, can cause serious illness.

Diabetes Mellitus

One might wonder why we will discuss diabetes mellitus in this super antioxidant book. There are two reasons. Number one, free radical damage to the beta cells that produce insulin in the pancreas has been implicated as a primary cause of diabetes. Number two, diabetic complications can be reduced drastically by the use of antioxidants.

Diabetes is a chronic disorder of carbohydrate, fat, and protein metabolism that is manifested by elevations of the fasting blood sugar levels. Additionally, the diabetic is at greatly increased risk for heart disease, cerebral vascular stroke, kidney disease, and the so-called diabetic neuropathy, where peripheral nerve function is dramatically impaired.

In diabetes, either the pancreas does not secrete enough insulin or the cells of the body become resistant to insulin; therefore, the blood sugar cannot get into the cells, which then leads to serious complications.

Presently there are approximately 5 million known diabetics in the United States and another 10 million who remain undiagnosed. There are basically two types of diabetes: Type I, which is an insulin-dependent diabetes mellitus (IDDM), occurring most often in youngsters or adolescents; and Type II, or non-insulin-dependent diabetes mellitus (NIDDM), which generally has an onset after the age of forty.

Generally the symptoms are the same, with the classic signs and symptoms of diabetes being frequent urination, excessive appetite, and excessive thirst. Other symptoms include blurring of the vision, itching of the skin, fatigue, slow wound healing, and skin infections, with associated tingling or numbness of the feet. Other indications of diabetes include lingering flulike symptoms, loss of hair on the legs, increased facial hair, and small, yellow bumps (known as xanthomas) anywhere on the body. Inflammation of the penis, particularly the glans and foreskin (balanophosthitis) often may be the first indication of diabetes mellitus. Tragically, millions of people lose their vision because of undiagnosed diabetes, and complications from diabetes are the third leading cause of death in the United States. A simple urine sugar analysis will detect unsuspected diabetes.

The exact cause of Type I diabetes remains unknown. However, a current theory is that injury to the insulin-producing beta cells in the pancreas, coupled with some defect in the tissues' ability to regenerate itself, produces diabetes mellitus. In Type I diabetes, the body's immune system apparently begins to attack the pancreas. This autoimmune disease is strongly linked to free radicals that damage the beta cells of the pancreas.

Ninety percent of all diabetics are Type II, non-insulin-dependent diabetes (NIDDM). In this particular case, insulin levels are elevated, indicating a loss of cellular sensitivity to insulin. Obesity is a key contributing factor here, with approximately 90 percent of the NIDDM patients being overweight. Most important, ultimately achieving a normal body weight is associated with a restoration of normal blood sugar in the vast majority of these patients.

The Biochemistry of Diabetes

Two important considerations. The first has to do with glycosylation, the binding of glucose to proteins that leads to changes in the structure and function of the body's proteins. In the diabetic, excessive glycosylation occurs with the proteins of the red blood cells, the lens of the eye, and the myelin sheath that surrounds the nerve cells of the nervous system. Glycosylation is not a good thing.

Secondly, the diabetic produces a by-product of glucose metabolism called sorbitol. It is formed within the cell through the action of the enzyme aldose reductase. In the nondiabetic, sorbitol is formed but broken down readily into fructose, another simple sugar. This allows the sorbitol to be excreted from the cell. In the diabetic, however, with frequent elevations in blood sugar levels, sorbitol accumulates in the cell and plays a major role in the complications of the diabetic.

The following diseases are linked to diabetes mellitus: atherosclerosis, diabetic neuropathy, diabetic retinopathy, diabetic nephropathy (kidney disease), and diabetic food ulcers.

The diabetic has a three-times-higher risk of dying prematurely of hardening of the arteries than the nondiabetic person. Therefore, aggressive risk reduction toward preventing atherosclerosis is vital. This has been looked at extensively in the section on cardiovascular health.

The loss of peripheral nerve function, with associated tingling, numbness, pain, and muscle weakness, are unfortunately too common in the diabetic. This diabetic neuropathy may produce impaired cardiac function (*i.e.,* arrhythmias), affect the gastrointestinal tract, affect the function of the bladder, and is commonly linked to impotence in the male. Evidence indicates that diabetic neuropathy is due to sorbitol accumulation in tissues.

Diabetic retinopathy is a very serious eye disease that can result in blindness. In fact, diabetic retinopathy remains the leading cause of blindness in the United States.

Diabetic kidney disease (nephropathy) is unfortunately a common diabetic complication and a leading cause of death in diabetes.

Finally, the problem of the diabetic foot ulcer remains a serious one. This is primarily due to the loss of blood supply to the extremity and the associated loss of feeling because of the peripheral neuropathy. Gangrene of the feet in diabetes is twenty times higher than in the normal population. Foot ulcers are, however, preventable through proper care. Avoid injury to the foot, and do not smoke. Well-fitted shoes and keeping the feet dry and clean and warm all contribute to improved foot care and prevention of ulceration.

The use of tobacco constricts peripheral blood vessels, resulting in impaired blood flow, which leads to gangrene and often amputation of the affected limb.

Supplements and Diabetes

The most important of all of the supplements for the diabetic is chromium. Many studies of the diabetic have shown that supplementation of the diet with chromium will decrease fasting blood sugar levels, improve glucose tolerance, lower insulin levels, and decrease total cholesterol and fat levels, while increasing HDL cholesterol.[9] Chromium deficiency may be the primary underlying factor contributing to the large number of Americans who suffer with blood sugar problems, both diabetes and hypoglycemia. Evidence is overwhelming that there is a significant chromium insufficiency in the United States.

Although a specific RDA has not been established, it is my recommendation that 200 to 400 mcg (micrograms) of chromium picolinate each day would appear necessary for optimal sugar regulation. Be sure to monitor blood sugar and consult your physician accordingly.

The Antioxidants, Specifically Vitamin C

The transportation of vitamin C into the cells is accomplished by its connection to insulin. Therefore, diabetics often do not have enough intracellular vitamin C, and vitamin C deficiency exists in many diabetics despite what would normally be considered adequate dietary consumption of vitamin C. This latent and chronic vitamin C deficiency leads to a number of the problems already discussed, including vascular disease, elevation of cholesterol (and its link to arteriosclerosis), and a significantly depressed immune system.

Very important is the fact that vitamin C in high doses (at least 2,000 milligrams per day) effectively reduces the accumulation of dangerous sorbitol in the red blood cells of diabetics.[10] Remember, the accumulation of sorbitol is linked to many complications of diabetes, particularly eye and nerve disorders.

Niacin and Niacinamide

Although not an antioxidant as such, niacin (vitamin B_3 or nicotinic acid), like chromium, is an essential component of the glucose-tolerance factor. This makes it an essential nutrient in the treatment of blood sugar conditions, both diabetes and hypoglycemia. Supplementing the diabetic's diet with vitamin B_3 has been shown to have many positive benefits (but take no more than 100 mg daily).

Vitamins B_6 B_{15} and B_{12}

Vitamin B_6 (50 to 100 mg daily) supplementation also has significant protective effects against developing diabetic nerve disease, or neuropathy. Vitamin B_{12} supplementation has been used with success in the diabetic neuropathy patient. Though 1,000 to 3,000 micrograms per day of vitamin B_{12} by mouth is considered sufficient, injections of vitamin B_{12} may be necessary, also.

Vitamin E

As we have already discovered, vitamin E is a powerful and important antioxidant. The diabetic has an increased requirement for vitamin E. Since it improves insulin action and exerts a number of other positive effects, it is recommended that vitamin E in doses of at least 800 to 1,200 I.U.s per day be taken.

Reduction of overall oxidative stress through the use of vitamin E supplements in the diabetic greatly reduces the long-term complications of diabetes. Finally, vitamin E also appears to play a role in the prevention of diabetes. One study showed that low vitamin E blood levels was associated with a four-times greater risk of developing diabetes.[11]

Zinc

Zinc is a potent antioxidant and an extremely important mineral in all aspects of insulin metabolism. It has a protective effect against pancreatic cell destruction. The diabetic typically excretes excessive amounts of zinc, and therefore requires supplementation.[12] It improves insulin levels in both the Type I and Type II diabetic and is very important in wound healing especially necessary in the diabetic.

FOODS THAT CONTAIN ZINC

- Brewer's yeast
- Egg yolks
- Fish
- Kelp
- Lamb
- Legumes
- Lima beans
- Liver
- Meats
- Mushrooms
- Oysters
- Pecans
- Poultry
- Pumpkin seeds
- Sardines
- Seafood
- Soy beans
- Soy lecithin
- Sunflower seeds
- Whole grains

HERBS THAT CONTAIN ZINC

- Alfalfa
- Burdock root
- Cayenne
- Dandelion
- Eye bright
- Hops
- Milk thistle
- Rose hips
- Skull cap
- Wild yam

The recommended daily dosage of zinc, preferably in the picolinate form, is 30 to 50 milligrams per day. Remember, more than 100 milligrams of zinc per day could depress the immune function and act in contrary fashion.

The Antioxidant Flavonoids

The flavonoids are very useful in treating diabetes. Quercetin promotes insulin secretion and along with other flavonoids is a potent inhibitor of sorbitol accumulation in the tissues and blood. The flavonoids increase intracellular vitamin C levels, resulting in less leakage of blood into the tissues, preventing bruising, and maybe most important, enhancing the immune system.

The diabetic should consider increasing the amounts of flavonoids in his diet per day and adding a flavonoid-rich extract, such as bilberry or grape seed. I personally take 200 milligrams of grape seed extract per day.

Garlic and onions have both demonstrated blood–sugar lowering potential. This seems to be linked with their sulfur-containing compounds. In addition to lowering blood sugar, garlic and onions have a very positive effect for the diabetic in that these two herbs of the lily family enhance the immune function, lower serum cholesterol, and de-sludge the blood, all of which are important in preventing complications found in the diabetic.

Exercise

In closing, exercise must be considered a vitally important part of any diabetic treatment program. Physical activity enhances insulin sensitivity with an associated diminished need for insulin. There is also associated improved glucose tolerance, and exercise has been shown to reduce total serum cholesterol and triglycerides and elevate the good-guy HDL cholesterol. Exercise encourages weight loss in the obese diabetic.

Finally, exercise increases the tissues' levels of chromium and the insulin receptivity in the insulin dependent patient. It would seem, then, that many of the beneficial effects of exercise may be related directly to improved chromium metabolism.

Glaucoma

Glaucoma can exist in an acute or chronic condition. The acute condition is a true medical emergency with dramatic increased pressure within the eye (intraocular), usually confined to one side. There is associated tremendous throbbing pain in the eye with altered vision. The pupil becomes dilated and ultimately fixed unless the pressure is reduced. Nausea, vomiting, and just systemically feeling terrible are common symptoms.

The more common form of glaucoma is the chronic glaucomatous condition. In this condition, there is a persistent elevation of the intraocular pressure (IOP); however, there are generally no signs or symptoms in the early stages. Therefore, intraocular pressures must be measured on a regular basis to determine this diagnosis. There is, of course, a gradual loss of vision, generally peripheral vision, which results in tunnel vision.

Glaucoma is caused by a greater production than outflow of intraocular fluid, the aqueous humor. This causes increased intraocular pressure. The normal IOP is 10 to 20 mmHg. However, in chronic glaucoma, the intraocular pressure in the mild to moderate form is up to 40 mmHg. In acute glaucoma, the intraocular pressure is even greater than 40 mmHg.

In the United States, there are approximately 2 million people with glaucoma, and almost 30 percent of these do not realize they are affected. Ninety percent suffer from the chronic type, and few family practitioners have ever seen a case of acute glaucoma. Glaucoma remains a major cause of blindness in adults.

The primary cause of glaucoma seems to be in an abnormality in the composition of the supportive structures of the eye between the content and composition of collagen, the most abundant protein in the body, including the eye. Here, collagen provides support to all the eye structures. Structural changes often reflect poor collagen integrity and function. These changes lead to blockage in the flow of the aqueous humor and the result is increased intraocular pressure.

A number of important antioxidants seem to be extremely beneficial in the prevention and control of glaucoma. Vitamin C is extremely important in maintaining collagen integrity.

Oral vitamin C beginning at 2,000 milligrams per day may be enough to control the moderate glaucoma problem. However, much higher doses (25 to even 50 grams per day) may be necessary in extreme cases. At times, intravenous vitamin C may be necessary.

The bioflavonoids, particularly the proanthocyanidins found in berries such as bilberry, aid in normal collagen metabolism and enhance the effects of vitamin C, improving capillary integrity, and stabilize the collagen matrix by preventing free-radical damage. The dosage of bilberry is 80 milligrams three times per day.

The citrus bioflavonoid rutin has also been shown to lower IOP.

Ginkgo biloba extract (GBE) standardized to contain 24 percent ginkgo flavonglycosides also has been effective in the treatment of glaucoma. The dosage for GBE is 40 to 80 milligrams three times per day.

Also, the condition of chronic glaucoma has been successfully treated through elimination of food allergies. In one study of over one hundred patients, exposure to food or environmental allergens demonstrated an immediate rise in intraocular pressure in addition to other typical allergy symptoms. It is obvious that food allergies should be investigated if you have been diagnosed with glaucoma.

Cataracts

Cataracts are a frequent complication of aging. The cataract is a cloudy deposit on the normally clear lens of the eye. In some cases, the cataract is small, grows slowly, and causes little problem, but in many instances the cataract grows to obscure the person's entire field of vision, effectively blinding the person. Normal medical treatment for this condition is to wait until the cataract is rather large, then remove the lens surgically. Laser treatment is not yet available. An implant is then used to replace the lens that was removed. It is quite common for cataracts to recur within a few years and this surgical procedure also raises the risk of macular degeneration.

Sadly, most of the websites for eye-care clinics that we looked at still say that no one knows what causes cataracts. This is absolutely false. Cataracts are caused by free radical damage. As melatonin production stops with aging, the immune and antioxidant systems are not as effective, and oxidative damage to the eye is unchecked. This free radical activity is most frequently caused by smoking, diabetes, radiation exposure (including sunlight), and the use of certain drugs such as cortisone.

The oxidative action involved has also been clearly identified as lipid peroxidation. We do not normally think of our eye lens as fatty, but it does have a fatty outer lining. The section on antioxidant enzymes in chapter 5 describes how lipid peroxidation works, but for now, let's just say that the body needs glutathione to wipe out the hydrogen peroxide. The problem is that patients with cataracts have significantly lower levels of glutathione in their blood. This means that hydrogen peroxide, which is a normal by-product of healthy cells, lies on the lens of the eye, grabbing the extra electrons it needs from the lens cells, thereby damaging the lens.

But the problem goes beyond that. Hydrogen peroxide also damages the DNA of lens cells when they try to replicate. This means that the new cells are not perfect copies of the old cells. They are a little bigger and irregular. They won't respond to growth stimulators and have lost the ability to reproduce. As years pass and this continues unchecked, the lens becomes misshapen and opaque because of the accumulation of damaged cells on the surface.

It is not likely that we will find a way to reverse the damage done in a person who has already developed cataracts—at least not in the next five years. So our focus must be on long-term prevention, and there is a great deal that we can do in this area. We already said that low glutathione is part of the problem. To produce more glutathione, we need to have more selenium, a mineral that is essential in forming glutathione. Melatonin supplements would be expected to help both as an antioxidant and as a regulator of other antioxidants. In both cases, supplementation should begin when the person is between forty and fifty-five years of age, long before the cataracts become an imminent threat.

Vitamin C was found to have little effect in one study, but apparently this study did not allow enough time. The more definitive study was published in the *American Journal of Nutrition* in October 1977, which followed 247 women ages 56 to 71 over a 10 to 12 year period. Among those who took vitamin C daily for a 10-year period, there were 77 percent fewer cases of early cataracts and 83 percent fewer cases that progressed to moderately severe. For women who took vitamin C for a shorter time, there was not any significant difference in the statistics. That means we need to be developing the habits that protect us from degenerative disease long before we begin to get sick—even before there are any signs of degeneration. It makes a big difference.

Vitamin E is also very helpful in prevention of cataracts, as it is in protecting all fatty tissues in the body. A recent study (*Ophthalmology*, May 1998) has found that people who take multivitamin supplements reduce their risk of cataracts by about one third. That's good, but those who regularly take a vitamin E supplement cut their risk in half! That's better. Being fat soluble, vitamin E is able to penetrate not only the lens lining, but the cell and nucleus wall to protect the cells from damage. It is quite possible that the main role of vitamin C in this disease is to rejuvenate oxidized vitamin E and make more of it available to the eye.

Two flavonoids have also been found to be effective in providing antioxidant protection to the lens. They are quercetin and quercetrin, both of which are found in the antioxidant complex Pycnogenol. These flavonoids block the production of an enzyme called aldose reductase, which is known to be involved in cataract formation.

Our recommendations for preventing cataracts are simply to implement an antioxidant supplementation program and stick with it. There are no short-term treatments. Cataracts take years to develop, usually in a person's fifties and sixties, so you need to be taking preventive measures for years before a problem has a chance to develop. That program should include the standards: vitamin C, vitamin E, selenium, and Pycnogenol or grape seed extract. Melatonin is also recommended to slow the effects of aging and promote better health into old age.

Macular Degeneration

Twenty percent of people over sixty-five years of age will lose all or part of their vision to macular degeneration. Those who live beyond age seventy-five face a 37 percent chance of losing their sight to the same disease. That means that, of the 30 million Americans currently over sixty-five, 6 to 11 million of them will go blind in the next few years because of macular degeneration.

So what is this disease? The macula is the part of the retina where light focuses after it passes through the lens and the eyeball. There are two ways in which this area of the retina can degenerate. First, the pigments in the retina that filter light are disturbed or absent, especially retinal purple. In this case, the light hitting the macula injures it directly and causes radiation-induced free radical damage in the macular cells. The second form of the disease is caused by a proliferation of capillaries around the retina. These capillaries can leak, which will cause the retina to detach from its protective lining. If they bleed, a mound of scar tissue forms, distorting the shape of the retina and gradually interfering with its nerve impulses. The first symptoms of the disease are decreased clarity of vision and distortion of shapes. As the disease progresses, the eye's light is focused more on scar tissue than nerve tissue and the central area of vision diminishes until nothing is left.

Like cataracts, the primary cause of macular degeneration is lipid peroxidation. We know this because the blood profiles of these patients show very low levels of selenium and glutathione but high levels of oxidized glutathione. That means that all the glutathione the body could produce was used up trying to fight off hydrogen peroxide, and there was not enough selenium to convert it back into usable glutathione. Their antioxidant system has broken down. In this case, hydrogen peroxide (singlet oxygen is also involved) attacks the walls of the capillaries and the lining of the retina, which is rich in fatty acids, compromising the integrity of both. It is highly likely that the capillaries have grown beyond their proper place because of mutations caused by oxidative damage to DNA. The net result is small blood vessels bleeding under the retina.

The only effective treatment of the condition is to use lasers to destroy the capillaries, but often more capillaries grow back, and the patient is no better off.

No nutritional therapy will remove scar tissue once it is formed, but we can reduce the risk of letting the capillaries degenerate in the first place. This will require some very specific antioxidants. Vitamins A, C, and E do very little to affect this problem. Some antioxidants work on specific organs or types of tissues, and we must use the right ones to get the job done.

To correct the lack of glutathione, we must introduce selenium. There is no other way to recycle the oxidized glutathione and return it to a usable form. This will bring the basic antioxidant system back to working order so it can deal with the hydrogen peroxide problem.

Ginkgo biloba is a key to maintaining the retina's capillary health. This herb increases blood flow in capillary networks, relaxes the capillaries, and also repairs oxidative damage to the capillary walls. It appears to repair damage in the retina also. When tested on people with vision already impaired by macular degeneration, a significant number of them were able to see better at long distances. If taken early as a preventive, ginkgo may help to avoid the problem altogether. I recommend 40 to 80 mg daily.

Bilberry extract is associated with improved eyesight in many ways. In particular, it is able to cross-link collagen fibers to strengthen capillary walls. It also plays a crucial role in the formation of retinal purple, the pigment that filters the blue spectrum of light, which does the most damage to the eye. I recommend 100 to 500 mg daily.

Carotenoids have been associated with a 43 percent drop in the incidence of macular degeneration. Specifically, the carotenoids lutein and zeaxanthin were identified as the most effective. Lutein is concentrated in the retina as no other antioxidant is. It fights free radicals there and also contributes to the formation of pigments in the retina. Zeaxanthin is formed by the body from lutein, and together, in the lens and retina, they absorb the ultraviolet light that reaches the retina so that it cannot damage the eye.

They are "nature's sunglasses." These carotenoids are found in dark green, leafy vegetables like spinach, collard greens, mustard greens, and kale. The best results were found in people who ate these vegetables five times a week.

Zinc is the most abundant mineral in the eyes, but zinc deficiency is very prevalent in the elderly. Apparently, zinc taken orally can slow the development of macular degeneration. Patients given zinc had less vision loss than those given a placebo after one and two years of treatment. Zinc is found in pumpkin seeds, sunflower seeds, soybeans, and meat. Daily intake should be 25 to 50 milligrams.

Macular degeneration does not happen overnight. It takes years for the condition to develop, so we have to start taking precautions *as early in life as possible*—even in childhood. Simple habits like wearing sunglasses and eating greens make a big difference later in life. The incidence of macular degeneration goes from 2 percent at age fifty-five to 20 percent at age sixty-five, so this would appear to be the most crucial time to stop development of the disease. The one habit to avoid is smoking. Smokers exhibit lowered levels of lutein and increased free radical damage as much as twenty years after they have quit smoking.

Your eyes have to last a lifetime. They are delicate and precise instruments, but they can withstand an amazing amount of abuse. The reduction of immune capacity associated with aging removes much of the eye's ability to recover from the strains we put it through. We must take care of our eyes early in life in order to enjoy them throughout our lifetime.

Alzheimer's Disease

Alzheimer's disease is a degenerative brain disorder that appears as a progressive deterioration of memory and mental function, commonly referred to as "dementia." In the United States, 10 percent of Americans over age sixty-five suffer from dementia of varying degrees. As many as 50 percent of these suffer from Alzheimer's disease. Alzheimer's disease has reached epidemic proportions in the United States. There has been a ten-fold increase in this century.

The disorder was identified first by a German neurologist named Alois Alzheimer in 1907. In Alzheimer's disease, mental deterioration progresses to such a degree that there is significant decline in the person's ability to function socially and at work. Memory and abstract thought processes become increasingly impaired. These are coupled with depression and disorientation, especially in the framework of time and space. Increasing inability to concentrate or communicate, with associated loss of bladder and bowel control, are common. In addition to memory loss, personality changes and severe mood swings also characterize this disorder. Ultimately the patient is totally incapacitated, and death usually follows within five to ten years.

The symptoms of Alzheimer's disease are believed to be primarily related to a reduced level of acetylcholine, a vital neurotransmitter that is especially important in memory function.

Although considered at one time to be a psychological disorder, Alzheimer's disease is now considered to be a degenerative disorder characterized by specific pathological changes in the brain. Here, nerve fibers that surround the brain's memory center, the hippocampus, become tangled, and information is no longer carried properly to and from the brain. Memories formed in younger years cannot be retrieved, and new memories cannot be formed.

Characteristic plaques accumulate in the brain as well. These are filled with an unusual protein, beta-amyloid, apparently a key part of this memory-destroying disorder. This substance is produced in virtually every cell in the body as a result of the generation of tissue. Although not itself highly toxic, it is probable that it is the trigger that brings on the dementia.

Although the exact cause of this disorder is unknown, high on the list as a potential causation is free radical damage and resultant oxidative stress in the brain.[13] Of course, it would make good sense as we age and desire to avoid this twentieth-century plague to increase our intake of antioxidants to cope with this oxidative stress.

There are a number of other interesting factors involved in Alzheimer's disease in terms of the cause. Many of the victims are nutritionally deficient. People with Alzheimer's have low levels of vitamin B_{12} and other B vitamins, which are extremely important in cognitive functioning. Too often, the type of diet of the elderly eat is made up primarily of man-made processed foods, from which much of the B vitamin content is removed. Zinc deficiency is common in the Alzheimer patient. Malabsorption obviously plays a significant role whereby normal nutrients cannot be obtained. Malabsorption is common among the elderly, making them more prone than others to nutritional deficiencies. Alcohol and many medications further deplete crucial vitamins and minerals.

As expected, many of the antioxidant vitamins, such as vitamins A and E, and the carotenoids (beta-carotene), are also low in the Alzheimer patient. Further deficiencies are characteristic of the Alzheimer patient: deficiencies of boron, selenium, and potassium.

Aluminum has long been known to play a role in Alzheimer's disease. Whether it is the cause or the effect is unknown, but aluminum accumulates in the brain of the Alzheimer's patient, where excessive amounts of aluminum are found in the hippocampus area and in the cerebral cortex. That area of the brain is responsible for the higher brain functions.

This excess aluminum may be connected to aluminum in our environment, such as aluminum cookware, antacids that contain aluminum, antidiarrhea preparations that contain aluminum, buffered aspirin that contains aluminum, and containers that are aluminum coated. Deodorants, food additives, and shampoos all contain aluminum.

Now, aluminum is not the only metal that has been associated with Alzheimer's disease. Toxic levels of mercury are commonly found. For what reason, we are not sure, but it could be related to the mercury from dental amalgams. It has been discovered that there is a direct correlation between the amount of inorganic mercury in the brain and the number of amalgam surfaces in the mouth.

Finally, another culprit in the death of brain cells is the immune system. The powerful immune system proteins called "complement proteins" have been found in and around the neurofibro tangles and in the plaques in the brains of deceased Alzheimer's victims. Experts theorize that complement proteins normally help clear away dead cells, but in Alzheimer's disease, they begin to attack healthy cells as well, and the degeneration of the cells results in accumulation of beta-amyloid. Evidence is also present that amyloid may trigger the release of the complement proteins, resulting in a vicious cycle of inflammation and further plaque deposits.

It is vital for you to know that the diagnosis of Alzheimer's disease, especially in its early stages, is very difficult and comes about only by a process of elimination. Although there are some characteristic changes on electroencephalograms and on the CAT scans of the brain, there is no specific diagnostic test for Alzheimer's disease.

One interesting note is that abnormal fingerprint patterns are associated with Alzheimer's disease.[14]

Treatment

Of course, early suspicion of Alzheimer's disease is very important. The sooner diet and lifestyle changes can be undertaken, the better. Avoid aluminum, especially that found in antiperspirants, antacids, and cookware. Diet must be improved to include more whole foods, fruits, and vegetables, especially uncooked, and less processed food and animal products. Supplementation should include high-potency multivitamins and minerals, especially the B complex. Injections of the B complex and vitamin B_{12}, in my experience, have at times brought about dramatic improvement. The minerals selenium and zinc especially are important as potent antioxidants. Zinc apparently helps stop amyloid plaque formation, which is related to zinc deficiency.

Other antioxidants to protect the brain should include vitamin C (2,000 to 6,000 milligrams in divided doses daily), beta-carotene, and vitamin E (400 to 800 I.U.s daily).

Doses are: zinc (50 to 100 milligrams daily); selenium (200 micrograms); the B complex injection (2 cc's of the complex and 1 cc of B_{12} three times weekly or more); acetyl-L-carnitine (500 milligrams three times daily); acetylcholine (500 milligrams three times daily); phosphatidyl serine (100 milligrams three times per day); and the essential fatty acids (can be taken from flax seed oil, 1 tablespoon per day).

Acetyl-L-carnitine is believed to enhance the brain's metabolism and slow the deterioration of memory. A deficiency in acetylcholine has been implicated as a possible cause of dementia. Phosphatidyl serine plays a major role in the integrity and fluidity of brain cell membranes. Under normal conditions, the brain manufactures significant levels of phosphatidyl serine, but if there is a deficiency of vitamin B_{12} and folic acid or the essential fatty acids, then the brain is unable to make sufficient phosphatidyl serine. Low levels of phosphatidyl serine in the brain are associated with impaired mental function and depression in the elderly.

One double-blind placebo-controlled multicenter study presented in the *Journal of Aging* in 1993 studied 494 elderly patients. Good results were obtained with phosphatidyl serine, improving the participants mental function, mood, and behavior.[15]

DHEA is the most abundant hormone found in the blood. It is found in especially high concentrations in the brain. DHEA levels decline with age, and many think that this contributes to the symptoms associated with aging, including impaired mental function. Declining levels of DHEA are linked to a number of conditions such as diabetes, obesity, elevated cholesterol, heart disease, arthritis, and other age-related conditions. DHEA has been studied in the area of memory enhancement and improvement of cognitive function. The dosage of DHEA should be 25 to 50 milligrams per day for men, and approximately half that for women. Individuals in their seventies and up may require higher doses. (See chapter 5, "DHEA" section.)

Ginkgo biloba extract, taken in either liquid or capsule form, is a potent antioxidant and increases blood flow to the brain. A recent study regarding this was presented in the *Journal of the American Medical Association*.[16] In this study, there was a dramatic comparison in the 202 patients with Alzheimer's disease who were treated with ginkgo biloba extract, as compared to the placebo, after one year. Ginkgo stabilized the Alzheimer's disease and lead to significant improvement in mental function in almost 65 percent of the patients. This extract of ginkgo should be a 24 percent ginkgo flavonglycoside dose and the recommended dosage is 80 milligrams three times per day.

In conclusion, it is my opinion that no one should accept a diagnosis of Alzheimer's disease without first undergoing a trial of intensive nutritional therapy, particularly the B complex and vitamin B12 injections. I personally have literally seen patients confined to a nursing home with the diagnosis of Alzheimer's disease treated in this fashion, and they dramatically improved and were ultimately discharged from the nursing facility.

AIDS

One of the diseases that has generated the most controversy and the most fear in the last decade is Acquired Immunodeficiency Syndrome (AIDS). As the name indicates, this is a disease where the immune system suddenly quits working. It does this when the human immunodeficiency virus (HIV) attaches to the receptor of CD4 lymphocytes, also known as T4 helper cells. The T lymphocytes are immune cells that help to trap and control foreign cells in the body. Typically, people don't die of AIDS, but instead die from a cold or flu that turns to pneumonia and other secondary infections because they have no immune ability to fight it off.

There are still many mysteries about this disease. One is that people can have the HIV virus that causes AIDS but show no symptoms of the disease until years later. Normally, it takes eight to ten years to progress from HIV infection to diagnosed AIDS. In about 5 percent of the cases, there seem to be no signs of disease after more than ten years. Why doesn't the virus automatically cause the disease? What makes it suddenly activate? It appears that the answer is related to the antioxidant capacity of the person. People with high levels of antioxidants in their blood tend to progress from HIV-positive to AIDS to fatal illness much slower than those with limited ability to handle free radicals. In particular, selenium levels seem to fall from extremely high levels, prior to the onset of the disease, to extremely low, and increasingly lower levels as the disease progresses. The section on selenium, in chapter 5, offers some insight on what might be triggering the virus to initiate the disease.

Chronic Fatigue Syndrome

Chronic fatigue syndrome (CFS) is an illness distinguished by feeling exhausted all the time, neurological problems such as vertigo or tunnel vision, and a variety of flulike symptoms. Patients often say it is like having a flu that lasts for six months, and just when you think you are getting better, you relapse and start over again. It is also known as chronic fatigue immune dysfunction syndrome (CFIDS), and outside of the United States is usually known as myalgic encephalomyelitis (ME). That's a mouthful, isn't it?

No one cause has ever been found for this disease, which is why researchers like Dr. Anthony Martin of La Salle University are looking for a cause related to free radical damage. Their studies found free radical damage to live red blood cells in people with the disease. Another hint of free radical damage is the immune dysfunction usually found in these patients. As you are learning, most antioxidants also boost the immune system.

Emotional and physical stress are known to make CFS symptoms get worse and are also prime conditions for ROS to flourish. Antioxidant benefits are multifaceted in this disease. They can reduce the damage to cell walls, especially of those red blood cells we mentioned. Antioxidants also protect the mitochondria of the cell, the cell's energy center and one of the most likely places to find free radical damage. The energy production of each cell relates to the energy of the whole organism or person. Antioxidants can also have infection-fighting abilities and antihistamine qualities that reduce the flulike and allergy symptoms.

Neurological Diseases
Parkinson's Disease

The distinct hand tremor, hesitant walk, and stammered speech of many older people are the classic signs of Parkinson's disease (PD). This disease is caused by the death of certain nerve cells that produce the neurotransmitter dopamine. These cells are in the section of the brain called the substantia nigra, and dopamine transmits the signals from this part of the brain to the next processing center. When there is not enough dopamine, the signals get mixed up and result in out-of-control movements. But what causes the brain cells to be damaged? It appears that this is one of the age-related diseases caused by oxidative stress, though there are other factors that determine why one person gets it and another doesn't. Recently, genetic factors have been found that may play a crucial role in the disease. But the actual damage to the nerve cells is related to ROS. The Mount Sinai School of Medicine found that post mortem studies in PD patients demonstrate increased iron, decreased antioxidants, mitochondrial defects, and oxidative damage to a variety of molecules in the substantia nigra. If the increased iron played a role in increasing the amount of oxidative stress, then it is likely that the hydroxyl radical was involved in the damage. Hydroxyl radicals are produced when hydrogen peroxide is exposed to free transition metals, such as iron and zinc. They are highly reactive and damage the first thing they touch. Three months after that study was published, a population study in the Netherlands found that people who took in more vitamin E, beta-carotene, and vitamin C were less likely to develop Parkinson's. The evidence was clear in both of these studies, but the news has not spread widely among those with PD yet.

Lou Gehrig's Disease (ALS)

Lou Gehrig, whose record of playing in 2,130 consecutive games stood from 1939 until 1996, was known as the Iron Man of Baseball. As a batter, he was overshadowed by teammate Babe Ruth, but usually had more RBIs and a better batting average than Ruth. As a first baseman, he was unparalleled, with a lifetime fielding average of .991. But only eight games into the 1939 season, something was definitely wrong. He only had four hits for the season, none for extra bases, and had been charged with two errors already, when that usually didn't happen until some fifteen or twenty games were played. Gerhig was diagnosed with a rare muscle-degenerating disease and forced into retirement immediately. His farewell speech, now immortalized by Gary Cooper's movie about his life, is one of the most touching moments in the history of sports. As he said, he considered himself the "luckiest man on the face of the earth." On that day, his number was retired and he was inducted into the Hall of Fame without the normal five-year waiting period. Two years later, he was dead. And the public was made aware of amyotrophic lateral sclerosis (ALS).

The name describes the disease pretty well, but only if you know Latin. *A-* means "no"; *myo-* means "muscle"; and *trophic-* means "nourishment." Together that means "no muscle nourishment." The word "lateral" refers to the areas of the spinal cord that send messages to the nerves that control the movement of muscles. "Sclerosis" refers to scarring, or plaque, that develops over an injured area. In this case, scarring over the lateral parts of the brain and spinal cord cut off the nerve signals to the muscles. No one has found a cause for the disease; there is no cure; and it is fatal.

The early symptoms may be so slight they are not noticeable: slightly delayed responses in the hands and feet. As the disease progresses, there will be slurred speech, noticeable weakness, and lack of coordination. In the final stages, breathing and swallowing become difficult as those muscles degenerate. The disease only affects the motor nerves, the ones responsible for movement. Mental faculties and senses remain sharp to the end.

There are three forms of the disease. The familial type is genetically passed from generation to generation. Another form is found with unusual frequency in Guam and the surrounding islands. The most common form here in the United States is the sporadic type, which seems to hit at random. The mutant gene has been isolated on chromosome 21. It is a gene coded for SOD, superoxide dismutase—the enzyme your body produces to destroy the superoxide radical. The defect in this gene results in an inability to produce SOD, which can protect the motor neurons. Other mutations have been found in the sporadic form of the disease. While this suggests some possibilities for treating at least this form of the disease, it is a long way from a cure.

Further research suggests that even mutant SOD still works reasonably well, but that it must be doing something harmful in addition to its reduction of superoxide. It now appears that it is peroxynitrate, not superoxide, which is the real culprit. The nerve fibers seem to be getting a nitrate coating by a mysterious process in which the mutant SOD actually helps the peroxynitrate attack the amino acid tryosine. Another process has been observed in which the zinc in the SOD molecule is actually extracted from it and joined with neurofilament-L, a protein abundant in nerve fiber. All of this is to say that we are finally making some progress toward understanding this disease, but there is no single antioxidant that will make it all better.

There is no evidence that suggests you can take SOD orally and use it in your body. Normally, it is produced all over your body and found in every cell. The problem in ALS seems to be that the gene that tells your body how to produce SOD is the one that doesn't work. Other antioxidants can be used to control peroxynitrate, such as OPCs from grape seed extract and Pycnogenol. DHEA has also had some remarkable effectiveness since its use with a few elderly patients, as reported by Dr. Alan Gaby in *The Townsend Letter*, but its mechanism is not clear. DHEA is known to be a hormone which declines with age and can act as an anti-aging agent when supplemented in later life. More research will be needed to find a definitive cure, but the advances in our understanding of oxidation and antioxidants have finally led to the only clues we have as to how a cure might be found.

New Kid on the Block

The latest research in treatment of ALS centers around a man-made polymer known as the buckyball. Its full name is the Buckminsterfullerene, named after the architect who designed a multifaceted spherical building for the Montreal Expo. Shaped like that building, the buckyball is a complex, all-carbon, multi-faceted sphere that acts as a "free radical sponge." Buckyballs are made by shooting a laser at two graphite rods. It has so many connections that it is able to give up lots of electrons and still remain stable. Its designers won the Nobel prize for chemistry in 1996. Laura L. Dugan at Washington University in St. Louis leads the research team that has shown these molecules can prevent nerve damage, delay the onset of ALS, and prolong life. No doubt it will have the same benefits for MS and Parkinson's patients.

Multiple Sclerosis

In contrast to the immune deficiency seen in AIDS and CFS, multiple sclerosis is caused by an overactive immune system. For some reason, the immune system in some people decides to attack the insulation tissue around the nerve cells called myelin. Myelin is very much like the insulation found in household wires and serves the same purpose—it keeps the electrical flow moving from nerve cell to nerve cell without being lost or interrupted. When the myelin breaks down, the nerve function does, too. When the nerve attempts to heal the damaged myelin, it produces scar tissue over the area. Hence the name of the disease refers to multiple areas of scarring (sclerosis) in the brain and nervous system.

MS is often said to be a little different in each individual, so it can be difficult to describe the symptoms. Some people diagnosed with MS never develop serious symptoms and others already have debilitating symptoms when they first see a doctor. Generally, the nerve damage affects motor control, sight, and cognitive abilities. It is also common for MS patients to have trouble sleeping. It affects mostly Caucasians, and women are more susceptible than men. It also seems to be almost nonexistent at the equator, but more prevalent as you move toward each pole.

The cause of MS has been very elusive. Many think that it is triggered by a virus, but they still can't explain why that would make the immune system attack myelin. While we haven't determined all the answers yet, the *Journal of Neurochemistry* has published several articles showing that much of the damage to nerve cells is caused by free radicals from nitric oxide. Normally, nitric oxide is a good thing in our bodies, but, when there is superoxide around, it turns to peroxynitrate, which is a reactive oxygen species. The scarred myelin is full of nitric oxide and some of it goes bad. When it does, the peroxynitrate attacks the mitochondria of the nerve cells and they can't produce the energy needed to carry nerve signals from one cell to the next. Their experiments, only published recently, showed that interferon-B was able to stop the nerve damage.

From what we know about antioxidants, SOD is needed to control superoxide. Since SOD is a ubiquitous enzyme, it should normally be attacking superoxide everywhere all the time. We need to find out why this superoxide is slipping by, but the real problem is the peryoxynitrate that it forms. We know that OPCs (like Pycnogenol and grape seed extract) will counteract peroxynitrate. No research has been done to confirm that Pycnogenol will have any affect on MS, but it is the antioxidant most likely to solve the peroxynitrite problem.

Another fascinating line of research indicates that the disease is affected by light and melatonin production. This can be a very complicated subject, and you need to read the section on melatonin for it to make sense, but here is an overview. When people are subjected to either low-level electromagnetic fields or natural sunlight (which have the same wavelength of radiation), they end up sleeping better, seeing better, speaking better, and having fewer bad days. This may explain why there is less MS close to the equator: The people in the tropics get more sun. Also, darker skin pigment (melanin) may be a preventive against MS. The key to this puzzle is that melatonin production both regulates nerve function in all these areas and acts as an antioxidant. Melatonin may be the missing antioxidant which allows peroxynitrate to attack the myelin. As a master hormone for the antioxidant system, melatonin may play a role in the production of SOD. If melatonin is absent, then SOD production may be cut back, increasing the amount of uncontrolled superoxides. One hundred percent of autopsies of MS cases revealed calcification of the pineal gland, which makes melatonin. Melatonin also stimulates serotonin, which enhances cognitive abilities and acts as a free radical scavenger to protect nerve cells.

Although research has not been directed to prove this, it would seem that supplements of melatonin and OPCs (Pycnogenol and grape seed extract) would be a reasonable response to address the oxidative damage in MS patients. Effective dosages cannot be determined without specific research, but they will probably be higher than the generally recommended dosages for these anti-oxidants.

Down's Syndrome

I know what you are thinking: "Down's syndrome? That's genetic, like a birth defect or something." Yes, there is a genetic basis for Down's syndrome. These patients seem to have some extra genetic material around chromosome 21, the same chromosome we mentioned in connection with ALS. In fact, the chromosome seems to be doubled. But even though Down's is caused by a genetic flaw, its progress is clearly related to nutrition and antioxidants.

Let's back up and talk about what Down's syndrome is. It is a disease that begins as the fetus develops, causing a complex of symptoms, from frequent sickness and poor muscle tone to mental retardation and premature death. The most notable outward sign in these children is a characteristic broad structure of the face and narrow eyes that has been called mongolism in reference to facial characteristics shared with the residents of Mongolia. Growth is usually stunted and there is a tendency to be a little plumper than others of similar height. The parents of these people know them to be very loving, affectionate, and joyful, which only adds to the tragedy of their short lives.

What that extra genetic material does is change the nutritional requirements of these children. That seems to be the cause of all the symptoms. There appears to be three or four times more ROS in DS cells than normal, and that needs to be controlled. Study after study has shown that given the right antioxidants, the symptoms associated with Down's syndrome can be slowed down or reversed. Given zinc, the thyroid begins working properly so that these children begin normal growth and their immune systems start functioning normally. Given selenium, their immune systems work better and they have more glutathione to fight against hydrogen peroxide. The problem of neural cells self-destructing is reversed when they have enough catalase (an antioxidant enzyme) or antioxidant vitamins.

One branch of research detailed how the genetic abnormalities led to specific damage to nerve and brain cells, resulting in retardation. What they found was that the brain does not develop with flaws, but that actions of particular amino acids and enzymes encoded in chromosome 21 allow ROS damage to the neural cells. Even as late as four months of age, the brains of DS patients have developed almost normally. But within the first year, atrophy has begun and the stage is set for mental retardation in life and Alzheimer's in adulthood.

There is clearly the suggestion here that the neurologic degenerative changes witnessed in Down's syndrome are not the congenital (present at birth) defects once thought, but rather, they are progressive, pathologic changes resulting—at least in part—from the genetic overexpression of SOD (superoxide dismutase). Further, if said neuronal damage is not congenital, then there may exist a window of opportunity wherein a specific intervention (*e.g.*, the judicious use of antioxidants) might avert the neuronal degeneration previously assumed to be unavoidable.

The implication is that the genetic mutation does not cause children to be born mentally retarded or having all the complications of DS, but it sets the stage for all of those complications to develop. Dr. Julian Whitaker, director of the Whitaker Wellness Institute, says that the basic mechanism at work is the overproduction of SOD caused by the extra gene. SOD is great at reducing the superoxide radical, but it leaves hydrogen peroxide as a by-product. It is the excessive amount of hydrogen peroxide that does the real damage. There are now some good indications that the damage can be reduced significantly by special nutritional supplements, especially if their is early intervention. These children need special supplementation beginning as soon as possible after birth and certainly within the first year.

Targeted Nutritional Intervention is a program developed by Trisomy 21 Research specifically to address the nutritional needs of DS children. The founder, Dixie Lawrence Tafoya, who has two children with DS, was profiled on ABC's *Day One* news magazine. She realized that her children were not retarded at birth, and she wanted to know what happened that caused the disease to develop. Her research led to the development of a nutritional supplement program that is receiving rave reviews. It is a broad nutritional approach that addresses antioxidant capacity, boosting immune system response, and building muscle tone. Those who have used this multivitamin and mineral supplement called Nutrivene-D report dramatic results very quickly. Children who have had chronic sinus infection all their lives are drainage free within days of starting the treatment because of improved immune responses. Appetite problems disappear, and growth, which had been retarded, suddenly resumes its normal progression. Motor skills, receptive language skills, and basic functioning are drastically improved. Of course, these results are considered "anecdotal," but research is under way to show the results in a scientifically acceptable form.

| CHAPTER FIVE

The Super Antioxidants

Introduction to Antioxidants

How Do Antioxidants Protect You?

Antioxidant defense system protects you at four levels:

- First, an *anti*oxidant keeps oxidants (free radicals) from forming. It also stops certain metals (*i.e.*, copper, cadmium, mercury, and lead) from initiating oxidation. What does this mean? Our bodies are like lead pipes. Expose a lead pipe to oxygen and it rusts; expose our bodies to oxidants and we essentially "rust" inside and our bodies break down. When a human body starts to break down, logically it is in a weakened state (the immune system is less effective) and we unwittingly open ourselves up to a number of degenerative diseases.
- Second, the antioxidant defense system intercepts oxidants (ROS) that manage to get formed and puts the brakes on chain reactions to stop the re-creation of numerous other oxidants. An easy analogy here is dominos. Once the first domino falls, it is difficult to catch all of the others before they go down as well. Once our body is in a weakened state and starting to degenerate due to oxidation, unless we take curative and preventive steps (eating foods rich in antioxidants and/or taking antioxidant supplements), it may be difficult to slow down or stop an oxidation chain reaction.
- Third, it intercepts damage caused by the oxidants that do not get intercepted. Your body is a truly marvelous thing! It has the ability to wipe out dangerous oxidants in your system, and then check and double-check to see that these toxins have been

eradicated. By keeping a sufficient amount of antioxidants in your body, you are helping it maintain its second and third lines of defense against diseases.

• Fourth, antioxidants eliminate and replace molecules that have been damaged beyond repair and cleans up after itself, removing undesirable substances generated by its activities. They not only fight and protect you against possible diseases and various forms of destruction to your body, antioxidants also clean up the battlefield afterwards.[17]

Antioxidants in General: An antioxidant is anything that destroys free radicals in the body. Three of the best antioxidants are vitamins C and E and beta-carotene, which have been proven to protect the body against oxidative damage. They are found in many types of foods, especially fruits and vegetables.

Vitamin C is the most studied antioxidant, so it should not be surprising that we know more about what it can do. Vitamin C boosts the body's immunity by strengthening the thymus and lymph glands. The best sources of vitamin C are tropical fruits, such as papaya and kiwi, but the more readily available citrus fruits, like grapefruits and oranges, are good sources of vitamin C as well.

Perhaps because of vitamin E's reputation of increasing sexual stamina, some people literally go "nuts" for it. All kinds of nuts, but especially almonds, are an excellent source of vitamin E, as are sunflower seeds. Cooking oils contain even more of this essential vitamin than nuts, but they are high in calories, and too much too often can lead to or add to a weight problem.

Orange and yellow fruits and vegetables are the best sources of beta-carotene. Try brightening up your meals with squash, pumpkin, mangos, and carrots in addition to green leafy vegetables like kale and spinach.

Beta-Carotene, Vitamin A, Vitamin C, and Vitamin E: These nutrients, known collectively as "protectors," provide the body with important antioxidant protection. These protector nutrients are the body's first line of defense against oxidative damage.

Can People Get Enough Antioxidants from Food? Many doctors doubt you can get enough vitamin E without supplements unless you consume too many fatty foods such as oil and salad dressing, but you can get the recommended 30 milligrams of beta-carotene and vitamin C in a healthy diet if you choose your foods wisely. However, eating enough of the right foods may not always be feasible for the elderly and other people who have problems with chewing, digestion, and absorption. These people should consider a nutritional supplement.

Amino Acids

Amino acids are normally thought of as the building blocks of proteins, but they are also crucial in the formation of many enzymes, hormones, and antibodies. They really play many roles in the way cells work, and their proper balance is crucial to maintaining good health.

Nutritionists divide amino acids into two categories: essential and nonessential. Those labels are really misleading. "Nonessential" means that, in the opinion of those who did the research, your body manufactures enough of these acids all by itself given a normal, balanced diet. Those chemicals that your body does not manufacture enough of they label as essential, meaning that it is essential that you go out of your way to take in extra amounts of these elements in your diet. Since the time this research was done and these labels were attached, we have learned a lot about the importance of some of those "nonessential" amino acids, especially as they relate to antioxidant activity. In some cases, the optimum level is now thought to be significantly higher than the researchers previously assumed, and the labels have been altered. For instance, cysteine, and tyrosine are now labeled "semi-essential" amino acids. If we ignore the labeling system and talk about which ones are essential to your health, glutathione, cysteine and alpha lipoic acid (ALA) have to be at the top of the list, at least in terms of what they do as antioxidants.

Alpha Lipoic Acid (ALA)

Lipoic acid may be the ideal antiaging antioxidant. It is an essential coenzyme factor in the production of energy and a powerful antioxidant on its own. Not only does lipoic acid improve your metabolism, it protects you from the harmful oxidative by-products of that metabolism.

Lipoic Acid Is "The Universal Antioxidant"

Lipoic acid can go anywhere in the body because of its unique characteristic of being both water and fat soluble. Because it directly and indirectly helps in the protection of every body component from oxidative stress, lipoic acid deserves to be called "the universal antioxidant."

Lipoic acid interacts synergistically with vitamins C and E, potentiating and conserving them. When your body is deficient in lipoic acid, the other antioxidants do not work as well together.

Lipoic Acid and Diabetes, Retinal Disease, Cataract Formation, and Peripheral Nerve and Heart Damage

Lipoic acid is good for the diabetic, normalizing the blood sugar, and even more important, protecting against glycation, which causes many of the disorders associated with diabetes. Used in Europe for decades, it is proven to reduce retinal disease, cataract formation, and peripheral nerve and heart damage. A dose of 300 to 600 milligrams per day may be necessary to control elevated sugar. If you take drugs or insulin, monitor your blood sugar closely. The normal dose as a preventive supplement is 20 to 50 milligrams per day.

Lipoic Acid Offers Protection Against Atherosclerosis

Lipoic acid can reduce elevated total serum cholesterol by 40 percent, as well as prevent the oxidation of LDL cholesterol, the oxidative reaction that results in hardening of the arteries. Lipoic acid is transported in LDL with vitamin E energizing it. Of course, vitamin E is the most potent antioxidant protector against LDL oxidation. Thus, lipoic acid offers double protection against atherosclerosis: It reduces total serum cholesterol and keeps it from oxidizing. Lipoic acid may improve oxygen uptake of the heart as well. It is just plain good for cardiovascular health and should be a part of all heart disease treatment.

Lipoic Acid Protects Against Cancer

There is also evidence that lipoic acid protects specifically against cancer. Oncogenes are genes that cause cancer. Nuclear Factor kappa-B (NF kappa-B) activates the oncogenes in the presence of free radicals and other carcinogens. This results in the unregulated cell growth of cancer. Lipoic acid can enter the cytosol of cells and prevent activation of the NF kappa-B. Additionally, lipoic acid enhances immune function, your first line of defense against cancer, by neutralizing free radicals that would compromise it. Again, lipoic acid is a double-barreled weapon against cancer, just as it is in protecting against cardiovascular disease. These are the two diseases that kill more of us in the United States than all of the others combined!

Lipoic Acid Is an Efficient Detoxifier for Neutralizing Toxic Metals

Finally, lipoic acid is an efficient detoxifier in that it binds up and neutralizes the toxic metals lead, mercury, and cadmium. Lead continues to plague us through auto exhausts. The very toxic mercury intoxicates us by way of our amalgam dental fillings and contaminated fish. Cadmium is present in cigarette smoke. Iron and copper are essential minerals, but excessive or unbound free iron and copper behave as free radical oxidants, a dangerous situation. As a chelator, lipoic acid controls these, too.

Cysteine

Cysteine is formed in the liver from homocysteine and methionine. It is a free radical scavenger that assists in the formation of glutathione. It stabilizes cell membranes and is helpful in asthma, smoking, and counteracting the effects of air pollution. As a chelator, it improves immune function and healing.

Glutamine

Glutamine, especially in conjunction with the antioxidant vitamins C and E, is a potent detoxifier at the cellular level. Glutamine levels fall with advancing age, and this decrease of glutamine in the aging population has been linked to a wide range of diseases, including diabetes and heart disease.

Glutathione

Dr. Richard Passwater states that "[w]ithin the cell where the real toxic war is being waged, the most important antioxidant is glutathione." This powerful antioxidant is a sulfur-containing tripeptide formed in the body from three amino acids: cysteine (a sulfur-containing amino acid), glutamic acid, and glycine.

"Glutathione Helps in Preventing and Battling Weight Gain, Hyperactivity, Alcohol, Sugar and Caffeine Addictions, Allergies, Arthritis, Cataracts, Lung and Skin, and Prostate and Bladder Cancers."

Glutathione helps both to prevent numerous diseases and, in doing so, to slow the aging process. Dr. Allen H. Pressman, in his book *The Glutathione Phenomenon*, states, "[g]lutathione helps in preventing and battling weight gain, hyperactivity, alcohol, sugar and caffeine addictions, allergies, arthritis, cataracts, lung and skin, and prostate and bladder cancers." He further points out that glutathione provides other health benefits including increased energy levels, enhanced brain function, and boosted immunity. A study done in Spain showed that frogs lived longer, healthier lives when given supplements of vitamin C and glutathione. In Dr. Passwater's preface to his book, he describes glutathione as "the foot soldiers in the battle against free radicals and toxins."

Half of Individuals over 65 Are Deficient in Glutathione, Leading to Greater Susceptibility to All Kinds of Disease, Especially Cancer

One of the key discoveries in understanding the importance of glutathione was that glutathione levels tend to be lower in older people. The decline in glutathione levels can be seen as early as age forty. At about that age, half of the population shows levels 25 to 30 percent lower than normal for the younger group. By age sixty-five, half of the people showed a deficiency of glutathione, leading to greater susceptibility to all kinds of disease, especially cancer. On the other hand, older people who have maintained high glutathione levels have longer, healthier lives with less occurrence of cancer. The realization that this one factor could explain the higher incidence of cancer in older people, various aspects of aging, and reduced immunity in the elderly and HIV patients has led to aggressive research into all three areas.

How Does Glutathione Work?

Glutathione is the key ingredient in neutralizing hydrogen peroxide in lipids and in the glutathione cycle itself. In the glutathione cycle, glutathione works with the enzyme glutathione peroxidase to scavenge hydrogen peroxide radicals in fatty tissues, such as cell membranes. When the battle is over, the hydrogen peroxide has been converted to water, but the glutathione is now in a disulfide form known as GSSG. Another enzyme, glutathione reductase, is then called on to reduce the GSSG back to normal glutathione so that the cycle can begin all over again. This is a crucial step in the antioxidant process. If it is not completed, dangerous hydroxyl radicals are formed.

In another similar mechanism, glutathione can attack an oxidant directly. In fact, if there are sufficient levels of glutathione, it can directly attack the powerful hydroxyl radical, converting it to water. The glutathione is then oxidized into GSSG, and glutathione reductase converts it back to usable glutathione, an amazing cycle. The reductase in this process needs to have vitamins B_1 and B_2 present for its activity. Basically the same mechanism is used by glutathione to protect cells from radiation damage. The fact that glutathione can neutralize hydroxyl radicals is very important. It means that there is a mechanism available in every organ of the body to handle this potent radical, *if* there are sufficient quantities available.

Over the Years, the Accumulation of Toxins in the Air and Water Pollutants, Processed Foods, and Chemical Exposure Takes its Toll on the Amount of Available Glutathione in Our Bodies—A Cancer Waiting to Happen?

Glutathione also acts as a detoxicant. There are at least twelve carcinogens that have been identified as being susceptible to attack from glutathione. When glutathione does this job, it bonds with the toxin and glutathione transferases to neutralize the poison, and then it leaves the cell to be eliminated in the bile or urine. For this glutathione to be replaced, more glutathione must be synthesized by the cell. If it is not able to do so, the cell is glutathione deficient and none of the things needed to be done by glutathione get done. This means that lipid peroxidation goes wild, other toxins can attack the cell, radiation damage is not repaired, and there is no regulation of antioxidant activity or DNA replication. In other words, it is a cancer waiting to happen. It is probably here, in the detoxification process, that we slowly lose glutathione with age. Over the years, the accumulation of toxins in air and water pollutants, processed foods, and chemical exposure takes its toll on the amount of available glutathione.

Replacing Glutathione Is Not Easy

Glutathione cannot be absorbed by the body intact. It must be manufactured in the cell itself. We can't even find a way for glutathione to move from cell to cell. Many people have thrown money away taking glutathione supplements that their body cannot use. In order to raise glutathione levels, we must give the body the components that it needs to synthesize its own glutathione. Glycine and glutamic acid seem to be readily available, but the limiting factor in the body's production of glutathione is the availability of cysteine.

The problem is complicated by two factors. First, cysteine is an amino acid that is rarely found in foods. Second, taking cysteine directly is toxic. However, the compound cystine can be taken effectively and it occurs in milk whey. Chemically, cystine is two molecules of the amino acid cysteine held together by a disulfide bond. When the cysteine passes into the cell, the bond breaks, leaving the cysteine intact inside the cell and ready to bond with the other elements to produce glutathione. A whey protein compound, called Immunocal™, has been developed that simulates the protein in human milk and delivers effective quantities of cysteine. It is not a drug; it is a food supplement derived from cow's milk, but with modifications that make it more like human milk in the proteins it delivers. Vitamin C also helps to keep glutathione levels up, but can't synthesize more glutathione, as cysteine can.

Recommendation

Remember, glutathione cannot be absorbed by the body intact. It must be broken down to cysteine first, then rebuilt by the cell. Many people have thrown money away taking glutathione supplements when it would be better to take cysteine and let your body do the rest. Vitamin C also helps to keep glutathione levels up.

Another approach to delivering cysteine into cells for the synthesis of glutathione has been injection or oral use of N-acetylcysteine. This method is also used as an antidote for acetaminophen toxicity. This does, at least temporarily, raise glutathione levels, but the side effects make it less desirable than taking cysteine supplements. Those side effects may include nausea, diarrhea, and anaphylactic reactions.

What Does This Mean in Terms of Fighting Disease?

Research has been done in the areas of aging, cancer, and HIV immunity impairment. In relation to aging, the decline in glutathione levels appears to be more consistent in explaining age-related disorders than any other antioxidant fluctuation. Moreover, separate studies have shown that Alzheimer's disease, cataracts, Parkinson's disease, and atherosclerosis are all either preceded by or associated with a decline in glutathione levels in the organ or systems involved.

As a cancer fighter, glutathione offers solutions to both of the major theories on cancer formation. Some believe that cancers are caused by exposure to carcinogenic chemicals, which may have a cumulative effect over time. But glutathione acts as a detoxifying agent specifically on many of the most common carcinogens, most notably aflatoxin B1. Glutathione also offers a remedy for the theory that cancers are caused by nonrepairable lesions accumulated over time and contributing to abnormal cell duplication. As an antioxidant, glutathione works to fight free radicals before they cause such lesions, it protects the mitochondria from damage, and it helps regulate DNA duplication to prevent cancerous cells from forming.

Oddly, there seems to be a higher concentration of glutathione in cancer cells than in the normal cells around the tumor. This becomes a problem in that it indicates that the cancer is using more than its share of glutathione precursors and leaving the other cells unprotected. But more important, cancer cells use the extra glutathione to protect themselves from attack, especially from the toxins used in chemotherapy. One reason for chemotherapy not working is that the cells have too much protection from their elevated glutathione levels. In a limited study, Immunocal™ was found to disperse these high levels of glutathione, allowing chemotherapy to be more effective, and boost the glutathione available to helper lymphocytes. So, if we feed the whole body what it needs to create glutathione, the imbalance seems to work itself out.

Glutathione's Importance to the Immune System

Glutathione's importance to the immune system cannot be over-estimated. The ability of lymphocytes to deal with oxidative damage can be measured directly by determining the ability of these cells to replenish their supplies of glutathione. This is especially true in the production of helper-lymphocytes CD4 and CD8 T cells. These cells are especially targeted by the AIDS virus, and a low CD4 count usually means that the disease is winning the battle. However, research at Stanford University now suggests that raising the glutathione level in patients extends their lives, even if their CD4 count is low. In addition, glutathione inhibits the replication of the HIV virus itself.

As if all that were not enough, glutathione also helps to maintain a ready supply of vitamins C and E. It does this by recycling these vitamins after they have been oxidized.

Methionine

Methionine has been determined to be a powerful antioxidant, a potent free radical scavenger.

Elevated Homocysteine Levels: Homocysteine is an amino acid that is intermediate in the conversion of methionine to cysteine. For those who are deficient in folic acid, vitamin B_6 (pyridoxine), or vitamin B_{12}, there will be an associated elevation of homocysteine. Homocysteine has been implicated in the formation of atherosclerosis, directly damaging the artery and affecting the blood-vessel wall, interfering with the formation of collagen.

Elevated homocysteine levels are a definite independent risk factor for heart attack, stroke, and other vascular disorders. Abnormal homocysteine levels are found in nearly 40 percent of patients with heart disease.

Taken from R. Clarke et al., "Hyperhomocysteinemia: An Independent Risk Factor for Vascular Disease," *New England Journal of Medicine* 324 (1991), pp. 1149–55.

N-acetylcysteine (NAC)

NAC Used to Treat Drug and Alcohol Overdoses; Also Tested as Treatment for AIDS

N-acetylcysteine (NAC) is the most common form of cysteine and extremely important in detoxification, often used to treat drug and alcohol overdoses. It is being presently tested as a treatment for AIDS because of its capacity to increase the T-cell lymphocyte numbers.

Cysteine has a protective effect against the development of oral cancer from the beginnings of leukoplakia. This is a particularly important supplement for those who smoke or chew tobacco or drink alcohol, leukoplakia being linked to all of these.

Cysteine is most effective when taken along with vitamins A, C, E, and selenium.

Soy and Amino Acids: Soy is the name for food made from soy beans, which are related to clover, peas, and alfalfa and are sometimes called soya. The beans are processed in different ways, making soy sauce, drinks, and curds. Soy is one of the plant foods that contains the proper balance of the essential amino acids. This makes it a valuable protein source, especially since it is low in fat and high in fiber.

Taken from Earl Mindell, *Super Antioxidant Miracle Book.*

Bioflavonoids

Stay with me here in this subchapter. You will be glad you did in the long run, but understand that you will be encountering some medical terms which may put your tongue into knots. These terms are "knot" easy, I know, but I will try to break them down for you along the way.

Diseases Known to Respond to Bioflavonoids

Allergy

Arthritis

Atherosclerosis

Bruising

Cancer

Diabetes

High blood cholesterol

Hypertension

Inflammation

Mellitus

Stroke

Varicose veins

Viral infections

Dosage of Total Flavonoids

The estimate average daily intake of total flavonoids in the United States is about 25 milligrams. An intake of greater than 30 milligrams significantly reduces the risk of cardiovascular mortality as seen in the Zutphen Elderly Study. However, when used for therapeutic purposes, a daily dose should be increased from 150 to 300 milligrams per day.

Polyphenols

What Are Polyphenols? Where Can I Find Them?

Poly what?

"Poly" is the Greek root for *polus,* which simply means "more than one" or "many." Polyphenols are "many" phenols that happen to contain a group of super antioxidants found in food. You may wish to incorporate many of these into your daily diet because of their powerful antioxidant benefits! Examples of several polyphenols are:

- **Flavonoids—5,000 identified elements that have super antioxidant qualities**

    Flavonoids—proanthocyanidins

    Food Source: red wine, bilberry, blueberries, purple grapes, feverfew, and ginkgo

    Flavonoid—citrus fruits—chemical elements such as pectin, quercitin, hesperidin and diosmin

    Food Source: oranges, lemons, berries, grapefruit

    green tea

    soy—isoflavone—chemical elements genistein, deidzein, glycitein
- **Resveratrol—powerful antioxidant that inhibits cancer cell growth**
- **Elegiac acid—prevents toxins from mutating genes, blocking the development of cancer cells**

    Food Source: strawberries, raspberries
- **Curcumin—blocks cancer-causing chemicals**

    Food Source: cumin
- **Cinnamic acid—anticancer properties**

    Food Source: cinnamon

Fruits, vegetables, and spices contain the greatest amount of flavonoids.

OPCs
(OLIGOMERIC PROANTHOCYANIDINS/PYCNOGENOL)

What is this one? Oli-good-gollie-what?

The main terms to visually recognize here are "Pycnogenol" and "OPCs."

Actually, the word "Pycnogenol" is a made-up word. It is a registered trademark. The term "Pycnogenol" describes an entire class of bioflavonoids that are composed of polyphenols or proanthocyanidin complexes. Pycnogenol can also be referred to as oligomeric proanthocyanidin complexes (OPCs).

> **Bioflavonoids**—"Bio" is the Greek prefix indicating a relationship to life. "Flavo" is a Latin prefix indicating the color yellow. "Flavone" is the chemical from which the natural colors of many vegetables are derived.
>
> **Polyphenols**—The term "polyphenols" (many phenols) is described above at the beginning of this chapter.
>
> **Proanthocyanidins**—"Proanthocyanidins" are a subgroup of polyphenols. They are flavonoids. "Anthocyanins" are any one of a group of reddish-purple pigments occurring in flowers.
>
> **Oligomeric**—"Olig" means "few" and "mero" is a Greek combining form meaning "a part."

Translation? Simply put, "Pycnogenol" = "OPCs" = groups of flavonoids

What is Pycnogenol?

The name Pycnogenol is a registered trademark of Horphag Industries in France and refers to a product they make from the bark of maritime pine trees (*pinus maritima*). This is a special pine tree found in the Quebec province of Canada and in southern France, located near the city of Bordeaux. Pycnogenol is both the name of a special class of flavonoids and a trademark that has two U.S. patents and other international patents. Dr. Jacques Masquelier was the person who coined the term "Pycnogenol," which also can be referred to as oligomeric proanthocyanidin complexes (OPCs).

Pycnogenol is not one chemical, but a complex of at least forty different substances extracted from the bark. All of these substances are water-soluble flavonoids that occur naturally in plants. The advantage of Pycnogenol is that it has a wide and important variety of many different micronutrients in one supplement. Pycnogenol is well absorbed and readily bioavailable, considered nontoxic, and is well tolerated. The name "Pycnogenol" was intended as a scientific name for this class of bioflavonoids, whether extracted from pine bark, grape seeds, grape skins, or cranberries.

According to Dr. Morton Walker, "Pycnogenol has been found to neutralize free radical pathology, which in large measure is responsible for such human difficulties as dysfunctional capillaries, bruises, malignancies, allergies, heart disease, peripheral vascular diseases, arthritis, varicose veins, diabetes, cancer, cataracts, scleroderma, multiple sclerosis, muscular dystrophy, Parkinson's disease, amyotrophic lateral sclerosis (ALS), and other forms of human tissue degenerations."

Pycnogenol is a great antioxidant, but that does not mean that it is a cure-all. Many claims have been made for Pycnogenol by marketers trying to sell their products, even though the research may not be supportive or the claims might be misleading. The research presented here is intended to clear the fog and stick to facts. No matter how good the antioxidant Pycnogenol might be, all the research suggests that we need a broad spectrum of antioxidants from a wide variety of food sources and that they tend to work synergistically in helping one another out.

The Discovery of Proanthocyanidins

Dr. Jacques Mesquelier discovered proanthocyanidins in a peculiar way. Upon a chance reading of the journals of the explorer Jacques Cartier, he found a story in which Cartier and his crew were marooned in the St. Lawrence River by the early arrival of winter in 1595. Being unprepared for winter in Quebec, their food quickly ran out, and there was an outbreak of scurvy that was killing the crew. A local Indian chief told Cartier that an infusion made from the bark of a pine tree would cure his crew. He tried it and recorded in his journal that his crew rapidly recovered. This story set Dr. Mesquelier on the course to find what could have been in this pine bark concoction. He knew that there could not have been enough vitamin C in the bark to do the trick, so he looked for something else. What he found was a mixture of bioflavonoids, including catechins and flavons, but with one particularly potent element called proanthocyanidin. He coined the term "Pycnogenol" to describe the mixture, took out a patent, and began marketing it in Europe in the mid-1950s.

What Does Pycnogenol Do?

Being water-soluble, it works primarily in the watery portions inside the cell and between cells, not in the fats of the cell membranes. "Pyc" is especially good at neutralizing the hydroxyl radical, the superoxide radical, singlet oxygen, and the dangerous chemical peroxynitrate.

The Dangerous Chemical Peroxynitrate

Peroxynitrate is a very reactive free radical that is formed by an overproduction of nitric oxide. Let's back up. Nitric oxide is usually a good thing in your body, helping with the regulation of some hormones, the movements of muscles in the digestive tract, and certain immune responses. It also helps the circulatory system by relaxing and opening blood vessels, stopping platelets from clumping together, and keeping LDL cholesterol from becoming oxidized. But sometimes the body goes overboard and produces too much nitric oxide. When this happens, the excess nitric oxide (NO) meets up with superoxide radicals (O_2-) and becomes peroxynitrate (ONOO). Remember Mr. Bill from the old *Saturday Night Live* show, saying, "Oh, NO-O-O!"? That's what we would say if we knew ONOO was forming.

What makes peroxynitrate so dangerous is that it reacts with anything: fats, protein, DNA, membrane, et cetera. It doesn't really matter what—peroxynitrate reacts! Excessive nitric oxide production is associated with arthritis, diabetes, stroke, septic shock, chronic inflammation, and atherosclerosis. The damage it does can easily lead to gene mutations, which replicate themselves as the beginnings of cancer. It can eat you up six ways from Sunday!

Good News! Pycnogenol Neutralizes Peroxynitrate

The good news is that Pycnogenol is great at neutralizing peroxynitrate. It also reduces the amount of superoxide available that makes the peroxynitrate and it helps to regulate the nitric oxide production so that it stays in balance. That means that your immune system works better, your joints hurt less, and your blood flows better, all because of Pycnogenol. Why didn't we mention this awful free radical before? The only research that mentions it is the information on Pycnogenol and other OPCs. Other antioxidants may help, but presently researchers have only noticed OPCs working on this problem.

How Does Pycnogenol Affect the Immune System?

Pycnogenol affects the immune system in several ways. First, it keeps hydrogen peroxide from combining with chloride (found in some white blood cells) to form hypochloric acid. When this acid forms, it is noxious—that is, it makes you feel nauseated—and it keeps your white blood cells from doing their job of fighting off disease. A 1996 study has also shown that Pycnogenol boosts the immune system. In this study, the immune systems of mice were blocked by infecting them with a retrovirus that causes mouse AIDS and/or feeding them ethanol. They measured certain immune system functions, then gave them Pycnogenol and measured them again. Researchers found out that immune stimulators were increased, immune suppressors decreased, and natural killer cells were stronger. In other words, even when the immune system was barely working, Pycnogenol brought it back. Research in this direction may be very significant for those interested in the AIDS virus.

Pycnogenol and Blood Pressure

Blood pressure can be lowered in some patients by Pycnogenol. There are enzymes in the blood that cause chemical reactions that make blood vessels constrict. That raises blood pressure. But Pycnogenol inhibits those enzymes, thus lowering blood pressure. It does not lower blood pressure a lot, but some. It also appears that Pycnogenol relaxes the blood vessels by counteracting the effects of adrenaline, the excitement hormone that is also found in stress cases. This is particularly important in the capillaries, where Pycnogenol has been shown to strengthen the vessel walls and open them for greater blood flow. Like the sprinklers in an irrigation system deliver the water, it is the capillaries that actually deliver blood and nutrients to the body cells. That means that every tissue in the body benefits.

Pycnogenol and Platelet Aggregation (Heart Attack, Stroke)

Platelet aggregation is a serious problem in cardiovascular disease. Platelet aggregation simply means that blood cells are abnormally clotting in the bloodstream. If platelets accumulate and clot in the coronary arteries near the heart muscle, blocking blood flow to the heart muscle itself, the result is myocardial infarction (the most common type of heart attack). If the same situation occurs in the brain's arteries, the result is stroke. Pycnogenol keeps platelets from clumping together, reducing the risk of both heart attack and stroke. A number of other factors cause platelet aggregation, including smoking and adrenaline surges from stress. Pycnogenol zaps the free radicals associated with smoking and blocks adrenaline to stop both of these factors from producing more clotting.

Pine Bark Extract May Help Immune System: Studies Confirm That Pycnogenol is Powerful, Protective Antioxidant: Pycnogenol, the pine bark extract that may help stimulate immune function, is a powerful protective antioxidant.

Dr. Lester Packer, a cell biologist and leader of a research term at the University of California who is studying Pycnogenol, declares that Pycnogenol contains about forty bioactive substances, many of which are antioxidants that neutralize free radicals.

Free radicals, of course, tend to damage white blood cells, reducing their ability in infection fighting, and their reduced numbers lead to inflammation and setting the stage for degenerative disease.

According to Dr. Packer, "[e]xperimentally, Pycnogenol turns off the production of nitric oxide, one of the major free radicals produced by white blood cells." He further states, "[b]ecause nitric oxide is also involved in inflammatory diseases, arthritis, diabetes, and heart disease, Pycnogenol should theoretically have some preventive role in these conditions as well."

According to Dr. Fabio Virgili, a member of Dr. Packer's research team, "Pycnogenol blocks enzymes involved in producing nitric oxide and directly neutralizes the excess free radicals."

In previous studies, Dr. Packer's research team discovered that

Pycnogenol neutralized other types of dangerous free radicals as well, including superoxide and the dangerous hydroxyl radicals.

Other studies have confirmed the immune-enhancing and antioxidant properties of Pycnogenol.

- In a study published in the journal *Life Sciences*, University of Arizona researchers report that Pycnogenol increases the activity of the natural killer cells, a type of immune cell that scavenges viruses and even cancer cells.
- Hungarian and German researchers have discovered that Pycnogenol reduces swelling and inflammation (this is from an article in *Pharmazie*).
- A study recently published in *Biochemistry and Molecular biology International*, a team of University of California researchers found Pycnogenol to be a powerful antioxidant against superoxide and the hydroxyl radicals.
- According to Dr. Packer, many researchers would want to break down Pycnogenol into its individual and active components. Dr. Packer stated, "[b]ut I think, in this case, Pycnogenol's collective effect [synergistic effect] may be much more potent."

The above research, which was gleaned from VERIS Research Information Service, was presented at the fourth annual meeting of the Oxygen Society held November 20–24, 1997, in San Francisco. This is an international organization whose members are scientists who study free radicals and antioxidants.

Pycnogenol and Atherosclerosis

There is also evidence that atherosclerosis has trouble developing in the presence of Pycnogenol. It prevents the oxidation of LDL cholesterol, which forms plaque when oxidized. Pycnogenol also maintains the health of the endothelium, the arterial lining. A 1994 study showed that blood vessels subjected to a strong oxidant (free radical) were not damaged nearly as much if they were pretreated with Pycnogenol. Cell viability was better, there was less evidence of lipid peroxidation, and fewer signs of tissue damage in the arteries. The reason was simply that the endothelium was protected from oxidative damage by the OPCs in Pycnogenol. If the endothelium is not damaged, there is no place for oxidized LDL to plant itself and the vessel remains healthy and flexible. Pycnogenol does double duty against atherosclerosis.

Pycnogenol Shown to Protect Arterial Endothelial Cells From Free Radical (Oxidant) Damage: Reactive oxygen species (free radicals/oxidants), such as superoxide and hydrogen peroxide, have been implicated in a number of degenerative diseases, including cancer, diabetes, and atherosclerosis. A number of antioxidant enzymes, including glutathione, catalase, and superoxide dismutase, play an important role in controlling these free radicals and preventing cellular damage.

Pycnogenol, a blend of procyanidins extracted from the maritime pine bark, have been shown to protect the arterial endothelial cells from free radical mediated damage.

Pycnogenol "[s]ignificantly decreased cellular accumulation of hydrogen peroxide following exposure to oxidative stress." The reduction of oxidative stress was dependent upon the Pycnogenol concentration. Additionally, Pycnogenol caused significant concentration-dependent decrease in the levels of the superoxide and ions as well. Further, the levels of glutathione, superoxide, and catalase were also increased in cells that were pretreated with Pycnogenol. "These results suggest that Pycnogenol promoted a protective antioxidative state by up-regulating important enzymatic and nonenzymatic oxidant-scavenging systems."

Taken from Z. A. Whei et al., *Redox Report*, Vol. 3 (1997), pp. 219–24.

Pycnogenol and Swollen Capillaries, Pain in the Lower Legs

Regarding capillary health, one of the common problems associated with capillaries is swelling (edema) and pain in the lower legs, especially in women. This is not life threatening, but it is a real concern that robs people of productivity and enjoyment of life. It turns out that Pycnogenol's effectiveness in strengthening capillary walls prevents leakage of water into the legs, preventing swelling and easing the symptoms of heaviness and pain.

Pycnogenol and Alzheimer's Disease

Preliminary studies show some promise in Pycnogenol's ability to fight Alzheimer's disease. Dr. Schubert at the Salk Institute in San Diego has shown that Pycnogenol can prevent an important contributing factor in Alzheimer's. The protein beta-amyloid normally occurs in the brain. However, in Alzheimer's patients, beta-amyloid accumulates and forms hard, scaly spots, in the brain. Pycnogenol prevents these accumulations, even when beta-amyloid is pumped into brain cells in a petri dish. There are also reports from patients having Newman-Pick's disease, which is closely related to Alzheimer's, that taking Pycnogenol has helped them. However, there are not enough cases and the studies have not been formalized to say that Pycnogenol reduces symptoms of these diseases.

Pycnogenol and Chronic Fatigue Syndrome

Chronic fatigue syndrome (CFS) has been a mystery disease for a long time and has been growing in its occurrence in modern times. It is now almost certain that the most basic cause of CFS is free radical damage. The damage is evident in red blood cells. Dr. Anthony Martin presented a paper at the 4th International Symposium on Pycnogenol in May of 1997 that spoke of five ways this antioxidant can help CFS sufferers. It protects the cell walls and it strengthens capillaries, as we have discussed. Both of these actions maintain integrity of the cells and organs and keep them nourished. More important, the mitochondria, the energy centers of the cell, are protected. If all the energy centers of the cells are healthy, the energy of the whole organism is enhanced. Pycnogenol also has anti-inflammatory qualities that relieve some of the chronic symptoms of the syndrome. And finally, it reduces histamine secretion, relieving the allergy symptoms commonly found with these patients.

Pycnogenol and Protection of the Skin from Ultraviolet Radiation

There are also benefits that Pycnogenol has for the skin. It reverses the oxidative damage done by ultraviolet radiation from the sun. With the ozone layer decreasing every year, more and more ultraviolet radiation comes through to the earth's surface. This is thought to be the cause of declines in frog, toad, and salamander populations, whose fertilized eggs are exposed to the sun with no way to repair the UV (ultraviolet) damage done to their DNA. In humans, UV radiation can cause sensitivity to light, capillary congestion leading to extreme redness of the skin, immune function changes, and cancer. Vitamin E has not been shown to be effective in reversing this damage, but Pycnogenol reduces the poisoning of the cell and lipid peroxidation in direct proportion to the amount taken. It also encourages the production of collagen and elastin, two substances essential to building flexibility and strength in skin and cartilage tissues.

Pycnogenol's Synergistic Effect

What makes Pycnogenol so great? Some scientists would like to break it all down and see exactly which elements make the biggest difference. But Dr. Lester Packer, a leading researcher in the field of cell biology at the University of California, says, "I think, in this case, Pycnogenol's collective effect [synergistic effect] may be much more potent." It is the way all of the different flavonoids in Pycnogenol work together that makes it effective in so many different ways.

You may have heard reports that Pycnogenol is fifty times more powerful than vitamin C as an antioxidant. Against some free radicals, that is probably accurate. The problem lies in the fact that we do not get to pick which kind of free radical we have in our bodies. We have them all! Vitamins C and E have proven to be more effective than Pycnogenol in other tests against other free radicals. It really depends on what you are testing.

Recommendation

Consider this as very important. The best course of action is to *use as many sources of antioxidants as you can* and let them *all* work together. Every antioxidant has specific functions and *all of them are needed* to fight the variety of free radicals that we must confront. I suggest a dosage of 50 to 100 mg daily of Pycnogenol.

Grape Seed Extract

The Key Uses of Grape Seed Extract: According to Michael Murray, a leading expert and author of *The Healing Power of Herbs*, the key uses of grape seed extract are as follows: 1) antioxidant supplementation, 2) atherosclerotic prevention, 3) capillary fragility and easy bruising, 4) diabetes, 5) retinopathy (macular degeneration and diabetic retinopathy), 6) varicose veins, and 7) wound healing.

Proanthocyanidins in General, Grape Seed Extract in Particular

All proanthocyanidins are basically identical, no matter their source, whether grape seeds, cranberries, pine bark, or others. The difference is in the varying concentrations in the different sources. Grape seed extract proanthocyanidin seems to yield the greatest concentration, at least 10 percent higher than that obtained from pine bark.

The product Protovin from Omega Biotech appears to be the most potent of all of the grape seed extracts, possibly because of the as-yet-unknown mineral content found in the grape seeds (possibly linked to the volcanic explosion in the Mount Saint Helen's epic some years ago). The grapes presently used in the grape seed extract at Omega Biotech are from this Washington-based vineyard. The exact HPLC studies done on other grape seed extracts have not seen the unique pattern present in the Omega Biotech samples.

Both the seeds and the skins of grapes contain proanthocyanidin, which is the molecule responsible for the protective and healing benefits. proanthocyanidin is a specific class of bioflavonoids found in a wide variety of plants, including purple, white, red, and green grapes, as well as pine bark, lemon tree bark, hazelnut tree leaves, blueberries, cherries, cranberries, and others. The most concentrated of these is in the seeds of the white and green grapes.

The French Paradox: The Antioxidants of Red and White Wine

The question is often asked: How is it that residents of France, who consumed such rich foods, have a low incidence of heart disease and cholesterol-related problems? The answer appears to be in their choice of beverage: red wine.

Following the harvest of the grapes, along with their stems and leaves, the grapes are pressed and the entire crush is placed in fermentation vats. During this process, the alcohol with the juice extracts the most soluble antioxidant from the grape seeds and skin into red wine. Eventually only the clear liquid is decanted into barrels and aged prior to bottling. The residue of the press, the so-called pommace, is discarded or made into lower-grade wines and vinegar. Grape seed extract from this type of material is consistently lower in value as far as its antioxidant potential.

The French Paradox: Paris (AP World News) 19 February 1998—"The French scientist who showed the world that wine is good for the heart has a new discovery. Two to three glasses of wine a day reduce death rates from all causes by up to 30 percent. Serge Renaud states in the *Journal of Epidemiology*, '[w]ine protects not only against heart disease, but also against most cancers.' His study of 34,000 middle-aged men living in eastern France supports what has become known as the 'French Paradox.'

"Frenchmen eat lots of saturated fats, but still live a long time. The results were the same for smokers, nonsmokers, and former smokers, he said. There were no differences between white-collar and working-class drinkers. In addition, recent studies in the United States found that a drink of almost any alcohol can lower death rates by reducing the risk of cancer disease. Renaud, however, maintains that wine is the answer. It acts against heart ailments in cancers because of its antioxidant action of the polyphenol compounds in the grapes (the OPCs or proanthocyanidins). He warns, however, '[w]ine is a more diluted form of alcohol and must be taken in moderation. After four glasses a day, wine has an adverse effect on the death rates and, although it still protects the heart, excess drinking raises the dangers of cancers and liver disease."

In the *Epidemiology* article, Renaud reported a 30 percent reduction in death rates from all causes from two to three glasses of wine per day, a 35 percent reduction from cardiovascular disease, and a 24 percent reduction from cancer. He is a cardiologist who works with the prestigious Inserm Unit at the University of Bordeaux. His book, *Healthy Diet*, is popular in France.

Renaud is also a strong advocate of the so-called Mediterranean Diet, based heavily on wheat, olive oil, and vegetables with more fish than red meat. And, of course, he adds a healthy amount of wine.

Red and White Wine Contain Antioxidants

Here is the basis of this French paradox. It is healthier to drink the red wine because this wine contains antioxidants that have been leached from the grape skins and seeds during the fermentation process.

In the production of white wine, the pommace is immediately separated from the juice following the crush. This separation prevents the leaching of antioxidants from the skin or the seed; therefore white grape pommace retains the best antioxidant, concentrated in the seeds, that when extracted produces a pink-beige powder.

Is the antioxidant derived from red grapes more potent than the antioxidant derived from green and white grapes? Professor Emeritus Jacques Masquelier, in the book *OPC in Practice* by Bert Schwitters, in collaboration with Dr. Masquelier, is quoted as saying, "[i]t is always a red pigment (anthocyanidins) which is derived from these colorless substances (proanthocyanidins). This transformation is produced spontaneously in nature in the autumn when the leaves of certain trees turn red. The differences between these pigments are fundamental as regards bioavailability and the effects on the human organism."

Well, what does all this mean? First of all, the coloration of red or purple grape seed extract is produced by two different factors. The first being the presence of flavons leached out from the skins and, secondly, the presence of anthocyanidins (red color) as a result of convertion from proanthocyanidins (colorless) in an acid environment. Further, the fermentation in the wine-making process provides the acid environment for this conversion to occur. Flavons are inferior antioxidants, so their presence does not contribute appreciably to the antioxidant potency of the extract. The amount of proanthocyanidins in the grape seed extract determines the antioxidant potency.

It is of interest that in almost all cases, the potency of the proanthocyanidin content is greater in the green and white grapes rather than the red grape; and since proanthocyanidins are the bioeffective antioxidants that produce the desired biological effect, it would seem logical to use the source that consistently produces the highest yield of proanthocyanidins, namely the green grape.

Laboratory analyses have demonstrated consistently that green grapes produce an antioxidant with higher cyanidolic content than those produced from red grapes.

Additionally, there has been no report of any superior grape species in the literature. Although some companies have claimed that they have a more potent grape species, this has not been proven in the laboratory or clinically.

Proanthocyanidins More Potent Than Resveratrol

Following is a comment about resveratrol, a known antioxidant, but one that has also been found to be much less potent than

antioxidants containing proanthocyanidins or monomeric catechins. In 1992, M. E. Cuvelier and H. Richard in *Biosci. and
Biotech Biochem* 1992 reviewed several papers that described the
chemical mechanism of the antioxidant effect of proanthocyanidins
and their building blocks, the catechins. These studies indicated
that the degree of potency of a particular polyphenolic molecule
as an antioxidant is directly proportional to the number of hydroxyl (OH) groups attached to it. Most catechins and epicatechins
contain five hydroxyl groups; some catechins contain six.
Proanthocyanidins contain ten. Resveratrol contains only three.
R. A. Larson, in *Phytochem* 1988 stated that polyphenols containing less than four hydroxyl groups show almost negligible
effects as antioxidants. Since anticancer effects are known to be
directly related to antioxidant efficacy, then proanthocyanidins
will be much more potent than resveratrol for this function. (NOTE:
Resveratrol is the supposed antioxidant in the trademarked product Procyanitol.)

In general, it must be understood that the analytical methods
used to assess product quality in terms of their biological activity
are not available yet. More clinical research is needed to discover
specifically which compounds are efficacious and bioavailable.
Methods will have to be developed specifically to measure this
activity. At present, no specific method of testing is available.

What Does Grape Seed Extract Do?

Grape seed extract does the following:

- It crosses the blood-brain barrier, scavenging free radicals
  within the brain.
- It protects against radiation, pesticides, chemical pollution,
  and heavy metals, all of which produce free radicals.
- It is assimilated into the body within seconds, enhancing
  the effectiveness of other nutrients in a synergistic fashion,
  such as vitamins A, C, and E.
- It inhibits the formation of certain enzymes that break down
  collagen and are the direct or indirect causes of allergies
  and inflammation. This inhibition prevents the production
  of histamine and thereby reduces allergic reactions.

- It improves the collagen matrix of blood vessels, thereby reducing leakage and improving circulation. Capillaries are able to carry more oxygenated red corpuscles to tissues, expediting soft tissue healing.

The Father of Grape Seed Extract Research

The father of grape seed extract research is the French scientist Dr. Jacques Masquelier, who, for the past fifty years, has been studying the proanthocyanidins. He was first put on the track of antioxidants by a fortuitous reading of explorer Jacques Cartier's journal, in which Cartier described the curing of his crew's scurvy by the ingestion of an infusion of the bark of a local pine tree. This pine tree turned out to be the famed maritime pine tree from which Pycnogenol is now extracted. Cartier and his crew had been marooned in the St. Lawrence River by the early arrival of winter in the fall of 1595. In a short time, their food supplies ran out and an outbreak of scurvy was killing the crew. An Indian chieftain told Cartier that an infusion made from the bark of a pine tree would cure his crew. He tried it and recorded in his journal that his crew rapidly recovered.

Masquelier was intrigued with the rapidity of their recovery, realizing that the pine bark contained only a small amount of vitamin C, which he was familiar with in terms of curing scurvy. He reasoned that the infusion must contain some other curative agent beside vitamin C and set out to find out what it was. After many years of research, he discovered the pine bark contained proanthocyanidins, and Masquelier coined the term "Pycnogenol" specifically for the proanthocyanidins derived from pine bark. He patented this extraction process and marketed the product in the mid-1950s in Europe; but because of the difficulty of growing and processing the pine trees, particularly the length of time needed to grow them, and because the process resulted in the death of the tree, Masquelier sought an alternative source of pro-anthocyanidins. His discovery was that proanthocyanidins were even higher in the grape seed. Most important, the grape seeds had a huge advantage over the pine bark in that they were not only quicker growing, but more readily abundant as a by-product of the local wine industry. Also, their harvest did not require de-struction of the plant. Although his initial discovery of proanthocyanidins was in pine bark, the vast majority of his research and work since then has been done on grape seeds. Even though proanthocyanidins are found in many plants, woody plants, and leguminous plants, the highest quantities are consistently found in grape seeds.

Proanthocyanidins Fifty Times More Potent than Vitamin E!

Proanthocyanidins are very powerful free radical scavengers that protect all of us from many damaging elements in our environment. These elements (free radicals) work against our immune system, our link to a vast number of degenerative diseases, and accelerate aging. The proanthocyanidins are the most potent of all the antioxidant protectorant nutrients, being as much as fifty times more potent than vitamin E and twenty times more potent than vitamin C. The proanthocyanidins have been studied extensively and have been found to be nontoxic. They are a group of the bioflavonoids known to be valuable nutrients supporting good health of tissues that are provided with abundant blood supply through capillaries. Capillary integrity is improved dramatically by the proanthocyanidins. They tend to affix themselves both on the inside and outside of cell membranes, especially the cells of blood vessels and connective tissues that are associated with skin and joints that contain collagen, protecting them from free radical damage.

Nutritional Benefits from the Bioflavonoids: Quoting Dr. Morton Walker from the "Medical Journalists' Report," 1991: "Although bioflavonoids are not true vitamins in the strictest sense, collectively they are sometimes referred to as vitamin P. Bioflavonoids enhance absorption of vitamin C and the two nutrients should be taken together. As synergistic agents, they are powerful antioxidants and free radical quenchers. Since the human body cannot produce bioflavonoids on its own, supplies of this nutrient must come from the diet. Food sources with appreciable quantities of bioflavonoids are not numerous. The following listing is of the best sources: grapes, oranges, grapefruits, tomatoes, rose hips, lemon juice, plums, papaya, cherries, apricots, and blackberries.

"Bioflavonoids assist vitamin C in keeping the intracellular cement collagen in healthy condition. They are essential to the human physiology because of their ability to strengthen the capillaries and regulate their permeability. This prevents capillary hemorrhage and rupture."

Grape Seed Extract Has an Anticancer Effect

Dr. Liviero L. Puglisi, from the *Journal of Fitother* (1994), pp. 203–9, regarding the antimutagenic activity of proanthocyanidins from *Vitis vinifera* said, "proanthocyanidins obtained from *Vitis vinifera* seeds were investigated in vitro for their antimutagenic effect. They resulted to be strong agents in counteracting spontaneous mutation, both at the mitochondrial and nuclear level of the cells. This effect, at least in part, is due to the antioxidant properties of proanthocyanidins and could be a rational basis for their potential use in chemo prevention of several pathologic situations (*i.e.*, cancer)."

Simply put, what this article demonstrates is that grape seed extract has an anticancer effect.

Diseases Positively Affected by OPCs: Here is a list of diseases positively affected by OPCs: Allergies, Arthritis, Atherosclerosis, Alzheimer's, Bruising, Cancer, Diabetes, High blood cholesterol, High blood pressure, Inflammation, Multiple sclerosis, Parkinson's disease, Stroke, Varicose veins, and Viral infections.

Back to the Wine

Now, back to the wine. Yes, the OPCs in red wine are apparently effective enough to overcome the effects of the high-fat French diet. Dr. Serge Renaud, a cardiologist at the University of Bordeaux, has studied the effects of wine for years, following more than thirty-four thousand middle-aged men living in France. He learned that the results were the same regardless of diet; smoking, whether the men were nonsmokers, or former smokers; and whether they were whitecollar or bluecollar. Those who drank two to three glasses of wine a day had 35 percent fewer heart attacks, 24 percent fewer cancers, and 30 percent fewer deaths from all causes. But don't go overboard. At four glasses of wine per day, there is a major reversal of the statistics and the death rates and cancer rates rise! At that point, the oxidative effect of the alcohol itself surpasses the benefits of the antioxidants. Socrates' maxim of "moderation in all things" applies once again. For those of you who cannot practice moderation in this area, don't use these findings as an excuse to ignore your disease: Get to an AA meeting, fast!

Dosage of Grape Seed Extract

The dosage for grape seed extract is approximately 150 to 200 milligrams per day.

Quercetin

Where is Quercetin Found and What Does It Do?

Quercetin is a potent flavonoid that is found in onions, cayenne pepper, garlic, and green tea. As a potent antioxidant, quercetin inhibits the production of free radicals (oxidants). In the cardiovascular system, it prevents free radicals from oxidizing low-density lipo proteins (LDL) or bad cholesterol. We have learned that LDL cholesterol, when it becomes oxidized, is the precursor to arterial damage and atherosclerosis, liked to coronary heart disease.

Quercetin has a positive effect on dangerous excess iron and slows the buildup of "abnormal-sticky" platelets in the bloodstream. Excess iron and "sticky platelets" are thought to be significant risk factors in atherosclerosis, which leads to heart attack and stroke.

Two large population studies are of significance. One, called the Zutphen Elderly Study, examined the risk factors of 805 elderly Dutch men aged sixty-five to eighty-four. Beginning in 1985, the researchers took stock of the participants' intake of quercetin and other flavonoids. In five years, the researchers tracked the participants whose major source of flavonoids were tea, onions, and apples.

It was found that the flavonoid intake decreased mortality from coronary heart disease and additionally decreased the incidence of the first heart attack. As expected, researchers also found that flavonoid intake was linked to a decreased risk of stroke by as much as one third of the risk factors.

The second study, called the Seven-Countries Study, took place between 1958 and 1964. Researchers followed 763 men living in Finland, Italy, Greece, the former Yugoslavia, Japan, the Netherlands, and the United States. Flavonoid intake was determined again to be associated with decreased death rates from coronary heart disease. Again, the protective effects of quercetin were associated with an increase in consumption.

Remember, the antioxidant quercetin is found in garlic, onions, cayenne pepper, and green tea. It can also be taken as a nutritional supplement.

FLAVONOID CLASSES—BASED ON CHEMICAL CHARACTERIZATIONS

Flavonoid Class	Class Members	Plant Sources
Flavonols	Catechins	Green tea, grape seeds, pine bark
Proanthocyanidins	Oligomeric catechins	Pine bark, grape seeds, leaves of bilberry, birch, ginkgo biloba
Flavones & flavonols	Quercetin, kaempferol	Apples, green tea, ginkgo leaves, grape skins, milk thistle, fruits
Biflavones	Amentoflavone, bilobetin	Ginkgo leaves
Flavanones	Hesperidin, naringin	Citrus peels
Flavanonoles	Taxifolin	Milk thistle fruits, pine bark
Anthocyanins, Anthocyanidins & Anthocyanosides	Cyanidin, delphinidin, malvidin, petunidin	Red and black grapes, red wine, bilberries
Flavonolignans	Silymarin	Milk thistle fruits, artichokes
Isoflavones	Genistein, diadzein	Soy beans

Carotenoids
Introduction to Carotenoids

Carotenoids are phytonutrients, and nutritional elements that give fruits and vegetables their distinctive colors, odors, and tastes. Although beta-carotene may be the best known and most abundant dietary carotenoid, approximately five hundred carotenoids have been identified, and their health benefits are beginning to be recognized. Carotenoids act as antioxidants, popularly thought of as antidisease and antiaging nutrients.

While free radicals can cause or complicate many diseases—including cancer, arthritis, cataracts, and heart disease—antioxidants can help protect the body from these chronic disorders. They also enhance the body's immune system.

It is also becoming clear that the best-known antioxidants (vitamins C and E and beta-carotene) do not provide a complete defense against free radicals. A combination of antioxidants works better than single antioxidants to enhance the body's defense against free radicals.

What are carotenoids?

Carotenoids are the substances that give fruits and vegetables their orange, yellow, and red colors. Green leafy vegetables are also high in carotenoids, but the color is masked by chlorophyll.

For many years the benefits of carotenoids were not known. However, recent research suggests that carotenoids offer an array of health benefits, such as lowering the risk for heart disease and certain types of cancer, enhancing the immune system, and protecting us from age-related macular degeneration, the leading cause of irreversible blindness among adults.

In addition to beta-carotene, a number of other carotenoids have been identified for their importance as antioxidants in the body. Alpha-carotene, for example, may be ten times more powerful than beta-carotene in protecting the body from skin, eye, liver, and lung damage. And the emerging body of scientific evidence shows that other types of carotenoids, such as lutein, cryptoxanthin, and zeaxanthin, may help protect individuals from certain types of cancer. In addition to their antioxidant properties, it's believed that carotenoids reduce cancer risk early on by their ability to enhance communication between premalignant cells and normal cells. The presence of carotenoids appears to result in normal cells sending growth-regulating signals to premalignant cells. Another carotenoid that has been identified for its health benefits is lycopene, a red carotenoid found in tomatoes and berries.

Does the average diet provide an adequate amount of carotenoids?

Carotenoids are not officially recognized as essential nutrients, but rather as a source of vitamin A. For this reason, there is no official RDA. However, the U.S. Department of Agriculture and the National Cancer Institute suggest one to two servings of carotenoid-rich foods daily.

How do I know if I'm getting enough?

There are a number of lifestyle factors that may increase your need for carotenoids. These include smoking, using oral contraceptives, and spending a lot of time outdoors where you are exposed to environmental pollutants and ultraviolet light. These factors can increase the number of damaging free radicals in the body, and therefore, people who are exposed to these risk factors may need more antioxidants, such as carotenoids.

To be sure you are getting enough of these important nutrients, eat foods rich in carotenoids. However, diet alone does not always provide adequate amounts of carotenoids. If you feel that you are not getting enough carotenoids in your diet, you may want to consider taking carotenoid supplements.

In addition, studies suggest that blood levels of carotenoids reflect recent dietary intake and are not indicative of long-term intake or body storage of carotenoids. Regular intake of carotenoid-containing foods or supplements seems to be necessary to maintain plasma levels of carotenoids.

It has also been suggested that taking large amounts of one type of carotenoid in supplement form may impair the absorption of other carotenoids. Thus, it is very important to take a carotenoid supplement that includes a variety of these important nutrients.

Information taken from "Carotenoids, Information and Facts" pamphlet put out by Henkel (1995).

Carotenoids in General (Alpha-Carotene, Beta-Carotene, Cryptoxanthin, Lutein and Zeaxanthin, Lycopene)

Folk wisdom has suggested for centuries that "the eating of color" is beneficial for health. Dieticians used to base their menus on the colors of foods, making sure there was a balance of red, green, orange, and yellow. This implies the health benefits in fruits and vegetables. Only in the past few decades have investigators recognized the many benefits of the pigments that give food their vibrant color. Carotenoids are a family of natural pigments found only in plants. There are more than six hundred carotenoids in all. Approximately sixty are found in foods and twenty are found in the modern diet. Evidence is growing that certain carotenoids are important to our health.

The carotenoids include alpha-carotene, beta-carotene, cryptoxanthin, lycopene, lutein, and zeaxanthin. These are all powerful antioxidant nutrients. Beta-carotene, alpha-carotene, and cryptoxanthin possess retinal activity. That is, the body can convert these carotenoids into vitamin A. However, lycopene, which is not a vitamin A precursor, has been found to be one of the more powerful of all antioxidant carotenoids.

Beta-Carotene: While each carotenoid has its unique benefits, mixtures of carotenoids, as found in a balanced diet, have proven even more effective. D. L. Morris presented an article in the *Journal of the American Medical Association* (November 1994) showing that blood levels of total carotenoids were related to heart disease. Of the two thousand men tested and monitored over a 13-year period, those with the highest levels of carotenoids in their blood had 40 percent fewer heart attacks than those with lower levels. Likewise, L. Marchand (*Cancer Epidemiology*, May 1993) showed that the lowest risk of lung cancer occurred in those with the highest intake of beta-carotene, alpha-carotene, and lutein. Many researchers have reported that mixed carotenoids protect the skin against the harmful effects of ultraviolet radiation. Additionally, if you take beta-carotene supplements, it seems to raise the blood levels of other carotenoids, too, indicating that it amplifies the body's absorption of other carotenoids (*American Journal of Clinical Nutrition*, December 1994). A mixed carotenoid supplement is made by Nutrilite.

Human Study—Carotenoids Can Reduce DNA Damage: In a human study, carotenoids were found to reduce DNA damage. Damage to DNA is believed to be the cause of most cancers. Much of this damage is caused by free radicals. Antioxidant nutrients, which include the carotenoids (beta-carotene, alpha-carotene, lycopene, and lutein) can quench free radicals and may reduce the risk of DNA damage.

In this study, scientists assessed the ability of specific high-carotenoid vegetables to reduce DNA damage. They measured the number of DNA strand breaks and the amount of DNA oxidation—that is, the free radical damage—in lymphocytes from twenty-three healthy men while eating their normal diets and after being placed on low-carotenoid diets. The men were then given daily servings of carrot juice, tomato juice, or a spinach-containing beverage each for two weeks. The researchers then measured whether these foods affected DNA strand breaks and oxidation.

The results of these studies revealed that each of the carotenoid-rich foods reduced the number of DNA strand breaks. Carrots resulted in a substantial decrease in DNA oxidation. Consumption of tomatoes (high in

lycopene) and carrots (high in beta-carotene and alpha-carotene) significantly lowered the number of DNA strand breaks. Spinach (high in lutein)
also reduced the number of DNA strand breaks, but not as strongly. A
substantial decrease in DNA oxidation occurred only during carrot juice
consumption, suggesting "[a] particular efficiency of alpha- and beta-carotene at quenching free radicals in vivo."

The implications of this study reinforce other researchers demonstrat-
ing the health benefits of the carotenoid family. These nutrients reduce
the number of DNA strand breaks and likely reduce the risk of cancerous
cell changes.

B. L. Pool-Zobel, A. Bub, H. Muller et al., "Consumption of Vegetables Reduces Genetic Damage in Humans: First Results of a Human Intervention
Trial with Carotenoid-Rich Foods, *Carcinogenesis* 18 (1997), pp. 1847–50.

Carotenoids — Beta-Carotene

Beta-carotene is the most thoroughly researched of the carotenoids,
but for decades was considered significant only as precursor of
vitamin A. This began to change when the U.S. National Academy of Scientists' diet, nutrition, and cancer studies recommended
that diets high in beta-carotene and low in fat would reduce the
risk of heart disease and cancer.

The More, the Beta: Some vegetables are richer in beta-carotene than
others, but when you mix them together you get not only a complete
dose of carotenes, but a tasty salad as well. One quick and easy way to
make a carotene salad is to puree and freeze a pumpkin. Then, whenever
you are in the mood for a salad mix, puree with some vinegar and oil,
garlic, and other herbs of your choice. Finally, pour the mixture over a
salad made up of your favorite greens and other vegetables and you have
a light meal or a healthy prelude to a main course.

According to the *Journal of Clinical Nutrition* (January 1991),
"One molecule of beta-carotene can quench up to 1,000 singlet
oxygen molecules." That's impressive! More important, it is one
of the few antioxidants that neutralize singlet oxygen.

Beta-Carotene, Rats, and Liver Cancer: Scientists fed beta-carotene
to laboratory rats before exposing them to a chemical known to cause
liver cancer. The results were that the beta-carotene significantly reduced
the number of liver cell DNA strand breaks caused by a cancer-causing
chemical. Beta-carotene also lowered the number of "chromosomal aberrations," which included deletions, fusions, and damage to the structure of DNA.

Taken from VERIS Research Information Service (1997), an article written by A. Sarkar, R. Basak, A. Bishayee et al., "B-Carotene Inhibits Rat Liver Chromosomal Aberrations and DNA Chain Break After a Single Injection of Diethylnitrosamine," *British Journal of Cancer* 76 (1997), pp. 855–61.

Beta-carotene has been especially effective in relation to cancer. J. P. Allard (*American Journal of Clinical Nutrition*, April 1994) showed that beta-carotene supplements reduce the number of free radicals in tobacco users. Just two months prior to that, the same journal published an article by Dr. Kumegaki stating that "beta-carotene supplements prevent radiation-induced free radical damage to chromosomes in human lymphocytes." Thus, free radical damage from two of the primary causes of cancer can be limited by beta-carotene. Further, beta-carotene has been shown to reduce the risk of lung cancer in nonsmokers and to prevent oral cancer.

How Does Beta-Carotene Fight Cancer?

Two mechanisms have been observed. The first has to do with cellular communication and the second with activating the immune system. In 1992, G. Wolfe (*Nutrition Reviews*, September 1992) showed that beta-carotene enhances normal communication between cells, called "gap junctions," while decreased gap junction communication is associated with cancer cells. The details of how and why this is so are still unclear, but the connection with beta-carotene is certain. Apparently the cells replicate more reliably when they can talk to one another better.

Beta Foods: According to the USDA, people need to include enough "beta" foods in their diets to get the recommended dosage. How much food would you have to eat to accomplish this? Any of these will do the job:

- 1 cup of cooked sweet potatoes
- 3 medium-sized carrots
- 3 cantaloupes
- 14 cups of cooked collard greens
- 23 cups of cooked broccoli

More recently, Dr. David Hughes (*Journal of Laboratory and Clinical Medicine*, March 1997), a researcher at the Institute of Food Research in England, showed that beta-carotene is very important to the immune system. In order to identify and destroy abnormal cells (including cancer cells), white blood cells must first distinguish them from normal cells. This is done through a protein called MHC2 that sits on the cell's surface and searches for abnormal cells. If one is found, the immune cells are warned and move in, attacking and removing the foreign cell. However, if the white blood cells do not have enough MHC2 proteins, the abnormal cells go unnoticed and the cancer can grow and spread. Dr. Hughes found that beta-carotene, and probably all the carotenoids, increase the number of MHC2 proteins and make the immune system more effective in their ability to initiate an immune response. "Our study found that beta-carotene can enhance part of the immune system that's known to be involved in tumor surveillance. This could be one way in which a vegetable-rich diet helps prevent cancer. Boosting the immune system in this way could also help to fight off infectious diseases, such as colds and flu." But Dr. Hughes also noticed that a chemical specifically made by the body to fight cancer (tumor necrosis factor alpha) was elevated in the subjects receiving beta-carotene. This gives beta-carotene a double-barreled attack against cancer.

The immune system also receives a boost in the activity of T and B cell lymphocytes, which help fight free radical damage. Specifically, levels of T4 and T8 immune cells improved with daily supplementation of beta-carotene. Even in HIV-positive patients, several markers of immune function improved, such as the number of natural killer cells and activated lymphocytes (*Journal of Nutrition*, March 1992).

In relation to heart disease, beta-carotene has shown several specific benefits. J. M. Gazeiano did a study using physicians who took beta-carotene supplements on alternate days. This reduced the risk of heart attack by 40 percent in the male physicians. The *Journal of Arteriosclerosis, Thrombosis and Vascular Biology* (June 1995) showed that beta-carotene inhibited the oxidation of polyunsaturated fatty acids, which contribute to coronary artery disease. It is these oxidized lipoproteins that clog and stiffen arteries, causing stress to the coronary system. An extensive study of twenty-five thousand men and women observed for up to fourteen years confirmed that the risk of heart attack increased as the blood levels of beta-carotene decreased (*Journal of Circulation*, September 1994).

Where to get which carotenoids: Here are the best places to get the five major carotenoids. The further along each list you go, the less you get. Your best strategy: eat them all . . . and more!

- **Alpha-Carotene**: canned pumpkin, carrots.
- **Beta-Carotene**: sweet potatoes, carrots, apricots, spinach, collard greens, canned pumpkin, cantaloupe.
- **Beta-Cryptoxanthin**: papaya, oranges, tangerines.
- **Lutein and Zeaxanthin**: kale, collard greens, spinach, Swiss chard, mustard greens, red pepper, okra, romaine lettuce.
- **Lycopene**: tomato juice, watermelon, guava, pink grapefruit, tomatoes.

Source: *Journal of the American Dietetic Association*, 93:284, (1993), chart compiled by Ingrid Van Tuinen.

Recommended amount: 10,000 to 25,000 I.U.s daily.

Vegetables—The Darker the Better: Dark vegetables such as spinach, broccoli, and kale are excellent sources of beta-carotene, as are collard greens, turnip greens, and beet greens. However, while you still get some nutrients and lots of fiber from raw vegetables, the amount of available beta-carotene more than doubles when you steam vegetables. Carotenes bind to fiber, making them harder to absorb. But lightly steaming the vegetables breaks the carotene-fiber bond and allows greater absorption.

Lutein and Zeaxanthin

The *Journal of the American Medical Association* presented a study in November 1994 by J. M. Seddon in which investigators at five U.S. eye centers examined the role of carotenoids in preventing macular degeneration. Macular degeneration is the major cause of blindness today and occurs when the macula (the place on the retina where light focuses) deteriorates. Nearly a thousand patients and controls were studied and the carotenoids lutein and zeaxanthin were found to give the most protection against macular degeneration. Dr. Kathleen M. Egan of the Harvard University School of Medicine has also presented evidence supporting dietary carotenoids' ability to protect older people from macular degeneration.

Zeaxanthin was found to block the activity of the peroxide radicals and consequently protect cell membranes from this and other free radical damage (*Journal of Biochemica et Biophysica Acta*, June 1992).

Lycopene

Who would have ever thought it? Spaghetti sauce, ketchup, and tomato paste can decrease your chances of developing certain types of cancers. Research at Harvard University involving nearly fifty thousand men over a six-year period revealed that those who ate these tomato-based products had up to a 45 percent less likelihood of developing prostate cancer. What's the secret tomato ingredient? The answer is lycopene, a carotenoid akin to beta-carotene, a potent antioxidant that contributes to the bright red color of a quality tomato. In fact, S. Franceschi wrote in the *International Journal of Cancer* (October 1994), "Dietary intake of tomatoes which contain high levels of lycopene appeared to protect against cancer of the mouth, pharynx, esophagus, stomach, colon and rectum in over 5,000 cancer patients and controls."

Although it is not totally understood, processed tomato products provide the most abundant source of lycopene in the American diet, and it seems to be more easily absorbed by the body when eaten in foods like spaghetti sauce, tomato paste, pizza sauce, and ketchup. Processing seems to concentrate the lycopene, and the small amounts of fat found in the processed products may increase lycopene absorption since it is fat soluble.

The Anticancer Properties of Tomatoes

The anticancer properties of tomatoes are being researched because of the well-known fact that prostate cancer is less common in the southern Mediterranean countries (Italy and Greece) where tomato-based foods are the dietary norm. (*See* the section on grape seed extract for more information about the Mediterranean diet.) Lycopene has been found to be even more potent than beta-carotene in quenching singlet oxygen, and researchers expect it to have a protective effect against many other cancers besides prostate cancer. For example, researchers at the University of Illinois report that women with the highest lycopene levels have a five-fold lower risk of developing precancerous signs of cervical cancer than women with the lowest lycopene levels.

Ongoing clinical research is now focusing on three key areas: lycopene's efficiency as an antioxidant, lycopene's control over cancer cell growth, and lycopene's specific role in enhancing communications between cells in human organs and tissues. Evidence is accumulating that lycopene has potent antioxidant properties that could well play a role in cancer prevention. Studies presented by Dr. Yoav Sharoni and Joseph Levy of Ben Gurion University in Israel show that lycopene is more potent in reducing cancer growth than either alpha- or beta-carotene, especially the cancers with fast-growing cells. It appears that the lycopene interferes with cancer cell communications so that both cell growth and cell movement were delayed in breast, lung, and endometrial cancer cells. They discovered also that lycopene increases cell differentiation, the process by which cells in the human body become specialized (*i.e*, become a liver, muscle, or heart cell, et cetera).

Lycopene Has Positive Effect Against Heart Disease and Cancer

Preliminary research by Dr. George Truscott of Keele University in Great Britain indicates that lycopene is at least twice as effective as beta-carotene in reducing damage caused by oxidation. A recent study by Dr. M. Aviram and his team at Ram Bam Medical Center in Haifa, Israel, demonstrated that Lyc-O-Mato™, natural tomato oleoresin, greatly increases the resistance of LDL cholesterol to oxidation. We know that oxidation is extremely important in the process of atherosclerosis. So here we have a substance, lycopene, which has a very positive effect against the two major killers in the U.S. today, heart disease and cancer. A group of scientists in Israel, using conventional crossbreeding methods, has developed a strain of tomatoes very rich in lycopene, with up to four times the amount found in regular tomatoes. In addition, they have developed a nonchemical process to extract the lycopene from these tomatoes.

Since the human body does not produce lycopene on its own, it is vital that people, especially smokers, drinkers, and others in a high cancer-risk group, be conscious of eating a lycopene-rich diet and strongly consider supplementation.

Lycopene and Myocardial Infarction (Heart Attack): Research has persistently suggested that oxidative change of LDL cholesterol accelerates the development of atherosclerosis. Most important in these various studies, antioxidant vitamins have been shown to inhibit this LDL oxidation and decrease the progression of atherosclerosis.

A recent multicentered (ten countries in Europe) study evaluated the adipose tissue concentrations of lycopene and its associated risk of acute myocardial infarction (heart attack). There was a significant inverse association between the fatty tissue concentrations of lycopene and the risk of first acute myocardial infarction. "We conclude that lycopene . . . may contribute to the protective effect of vegetable consumption on myocardial infarction risk."

Taken from L. Kohlmeier et al., *American Journal of Epidemiology* 146 (1997), pp. 618–26.

Lycopene and Cancer Prevention in the Prostate

Lycopene is the most abundant carotenoid present in human plasma and tissues. Lycopene is especially highly concentrated in the prostate and undoubtedly has a protective benefit to the prostate as an antioxidant. Oxidative stress is always identified in the prostate tissue that develops into malignant cancer. The oxidation caused by free radicals damages the proteins and the DNA by chemically altering them. The magnitude of this oxidative damage increases with age, as does the incidence of prostate cancer. Studies have indicated that the antioxidants vitamin E, selenium, and lycopene all reduce the risk of prostate cancer. Therefore, it would seem that lycopene is extremely important in the overall role of cancer prevention in the prostate.

A growing body of scientific evidence indicates that lycopene is an important part of the human organism's defense against harmful free radicals, which are the major cause of numerous degenerative diseases. Scientists associate this property to lycopene's long-chain molecular structure, which contains thirteen double bonds, more than any other carotenoid. This unique double-bonded character is very important in its function as an antioxidant, being able to neutralize free radicals easily. Although not created by the human body, findings indicate that lycopene is an important part of the human organism's defense mechanism against oxidative agents, especially singlet oxygen.

Recent studies have shown that the bioavailability and protective effect of lycopene is enhanced by the presence of other natural antioxidants, such as the tocopherols and beta-carotene. In fact, one study attempted to use beta-carotene alone to fight

cancer and failed miserably. Researchers learned an important les-
son that just because a diet rich in certain foods may reduce cancer risk, isolating the compounds in that food may not have the
same effect. The beneficial chemicals in foods like beta-carotene
work in concert, in synergy, making the surest route to good health
eating whole foods and not some extract of them. Dr. Gary R.
Beecher points out,

> [t]omatoes are not just repositories of lycopene, they are also
> rich sources of essential nutrients such as vitamin C, potassium,
> folic acid as well as beta-carotene. Other flavonoids and
> phytonutrients, all of which may be related to the health benefit
> of tomatoes, must be studied also. This synergy within this lyco-
> pene—Lyc-O-Mato™ product may be the reason for its remark-
> able success against cancer and other oxidative stress disorders.

In a recent article in the *American Journal of Epidemiology*
(1997), Lenore Kohlmeier, et al., presented a multicentered case
control study to evaluate the relation between antioxidant status, assessed by biomarkers, and acute myocardial infarction. In
this study, a post-tissue needle-aspiration biopsy was taken
shortly after the myocardial infarction and analyzed for carotenoids and tocopherols. Lycopene was the only carotenoid that
seemed to be independently protective of myocardial infarction.
This helped explain why vegetable consumption seems to reduce the risk of heart attack. This study came about because
scientists are beginning to understand that lipid metabolism and
oxidation of low-density lipoproteins accelerate atherogenesis
and that supplementation of the antioxidant vitamin E, lycopene, and other bioflavonoids reduce the incidence of nonfatal
myocardial infarction. It was hypothesized in this study that
natural antioxidants present in the diet might inhibit the oxidative modification of LDL cholesterol and thus slow the progression of atherosclerosis. However, several large-scale trials have
not confirmed a protective effect of beta-carotene and are in-
consistent for vitamin E.

Since lycopene is a fat-soluble substance, Dr. John W. Erdman
of the University of Illinois in Chicago states, "If it is to be absorbed through the intestines, it must be consumed with some
fat. In fact, drinking tomato juice by itself may result in no mean-

ingful absorption of lycopene." For best results, lycopene and fat should be some part of the same meal.

Contrary to naturopathic thinking, cooking seems to enhance the available lycopene in tomatoes by breaking down fibrous cell walls that inhibit its release from the raw food. Thus, lycopene from processed tomato products such as sauce, salsa, paste, ketchup, soup, and canned tomatoes is likely to be better absorbed than that from a raw tomato.

The season in which a fruit or vegetable containing carotenoids is grown affects how much pigment it contains. A 1996 study done in the United Kingdom examined differences in beta-carotene, lycopene, and lutein content from foods grown in different seasons. The results indicated that it is extremely difficult to consistently achieve recommended daily amounts of carotenoids year round. However, protection against free radicals is necessary daily all the year through.

Additionally, preserved foods, both canned and frozen, contained significantly less total carotenoid content than fresh foods. But fresh does not always mean better. Giovannuci's study showed that cooked tomatoes and tomato products are better at preventing prostate cancer than uncooked tomatoes. In this case, cooking seems to make the lycopene more available, especially when a touch of oil is added.

Recommendation

Most important is that all of the carotenoids are very bioavailable in supplementary form. In my opinion, nutritional supplementation with antioxidants that include mixed carotenoids is a wise measure that can improve the odds of a longer and healthier life.

CAROTENOID CONTENT OF FRUITS AND VEGETABLES
microgram/ounce (1 gram = 1 million micrograms)

Fruit or vegetable	beta-carotene	alpha-carotene	lutein & zeaxanthin	lycopene	cryptoxanthin
Apple, raw	7	0	13	0	0
Apricot, canned, drained	425	0	1	18	0
Apricot, dried	4,990	0	0	245	0
Apricot, raw	999	0	1	0	0
Asparagus, raw	127	3	181	0	0

Fruit or vegetable	beta-carotene	alpha-carotene	lutein & zeaxanthin	lycopene	cryptoxanthin
Avocado, raw	10	0	91	0	0
Banana, raw	0	0	0	18	0
Basil, not dried	99	0	0	245	0
Beet greens	726	0.9	2,183	0	0
Beets, canned	0.3	0	1	0	0
Bitter melon, raw	14	0	0	0	0
Blueberries	4	0	10	0	0
Bottle gourd, raw	1	0	0	0	0
Broccoli, cooked	369	0.3	510	0	0
Broccoli, raw	198	0.3	539	0	0
Brussels sprouts	136	2	369	0	0
Cabbage, Chinese, raw	18	0.3	11	0	0
Cabbage, Chinese, wild	150	0	0	0	0
Cabbage, red, raw	4	0.3	7	0	0
Cabbage, white	23	0	43	0	0
Cantaloupe	851	10	0	0	0
Carrot,cooked, canned, frozen	2,778	1,049	74	0	0
Carrot, raw	2,240	1,021	74	0	0
Carrot A+ variety, raw	5,174	3,019	0	0	0
Carrot A+ variety, cooked	7,272	4,253	0	0	0
Cashew apple, raw	44	4	0	0	0
Cashew apple, juice	23	0	0	14	14
Cassava leaf	851	0	0	0	0
Cauliflower	2	0	9	0	0
Celeriac, raw	0	0	0.3	0	0
Celery	201	0	1,021	0	0
Chicory leaf, raw	972	0	2,920	0	0
Coriander, not dried	567	0	0	0	0
Corn, yellow	14	14	221	0	0
Cranberries, raw	6	0.3	8	0	0
Cress leaf, raw	1,177	0	3,544	0	0
Cucumber pickle	51	0	145	0	0
Cucumber, raw	2	0	68	0	0
Currants, raw	18	0	68	0	0
Dill, not dried	1,276	0	1,899	0	0
Eggplant	10	0	0	0	0
Endive	369	0	1,134	0	0
Fennel leaves	1,259	0	0	0	0
Grapefruit, pink, raw	371	0	0	953	0
Grapefruit, white, raw	4	0.3	3	0	0
Grapes, raw	9	0.3	20	0	0
Green beans	179	12	210	0	0
Greens, collard	1,531	0	4,621	0	0
Greens, fiddlehead	553	79	0	0	0

Fruit or vegetable	beta-carotene	alpha-carotene	lutein & zeaxanthin	lycopene	cryptoxanthin
Greens, mustard	765	0	2,807	0	0
Guava juice	77	7	6,209	947	0
Guava, raw	230	20	0	1,531	0
Jackfruit, raw	7	0	0	0	0
Jellies, jams, preserves	5	0	2	0	0
Kale	1,332	0	6,209	0	0
Kale, Chinese	40	0	0	0	0
Kiwi fruit, raw	12	0	51	0	0
Leek, raw	284	0	539	0	0
Lemon, raw	1	0	3	0	0
Lettuce, iceberg	136	0	397	0	0
Lettuce, leaf	340	0.3	510	0	0
Lettuce, romaine	539	0	1,616	0	0
Lima beans, cooked	0	0	0	0	0
Loofah fruit, raw	13	0	0	0	0
Mango, raw	369	0	0	0	15
Mint, not dried	213	0	0	0	0
Mushroom	0	0	0	0	0
Nectarine, raw	29	0	4	0	12
Okra, raw	48	8	1,928	0	0
Olive, green	79	0	145	0	5
Onion, yellow, raw	45	0	5	0	0
Orange juice	2	2	21	0	7
Orange, raw	11	6	4	0	42
Papaya, raw	28	0	0	0	133
Parsley, not dried	1,503	0	2,892	0	0
Peach, canned, drained	28	0	8	0	13
Peach, dried	2,624	0	53	0	71
Peach, raw	28	0.3	4	0	0
Pear, raw	5	0	31	0	12
Peas, green	99	5	482	0	0
Pepper, green, raw	65	3	198	0	0
Pepper, red	624	17	1,928	0	0
Pepper, yellow, raw	43	26	218	0	0
Pigeon peas	11	0	0	0	0
Pineapple, canned, drained	5	0.3	1	0	0
Plum, raw	122	0	68	0	0
Potato salad	3	1	0	0	0
Potato, white, cooked	0	0	0	0	0
Potato, white, raw	2	0	10	0	0
Prune, dried	40	9	34	0	0
Pumpkin	879	1,077	425	0	0
Radish, red	3	0	3	0	0
Raisins	0	0	0.3	0	0
Raspberries, raw	2	2	22	0	0
Rhubarb, raw	17	0	48	0	0
Roquette, raw	981	0	0	0	0

Fruit or vegetable	beta-carotene	alpha-carotene	lutein & zeaxanthin	lycopene	cryptoxanthin
Rose hip, puree, canned	119	0	0	221	0
Rutabaga, raw	0.3	0	0	0	0
Scallion, raw	241	0	0	595	0
Spinach, cooked	1,559	0	3,572	0	0
Spinach, raw	1,162	0	2,892	0	0
Squash, summer	119	3	340	0	0
Squash, winter, cooked	680	3	11	0	0
Squash, summer, raw	232	3	11	0	0
Strawberries	3	1	9	0	0
Sweet potato, cooked	2,495	0	0	0	0
Sweet potato, raw	2,523	0	0	0	0
Swiss chard, raw	1,034	13	3,119	0	0
Tangerine, tangelo juice	2	1	38	0	61
Tangerine, raw	11	6	6	0	30
Tomato juice, canned	255	0	94	2,432	0
Tomato paste, canned	482	0	54	1,843	0
Tomato sauce, canned	284	0	12	0	0
Tomato, raw	147	0	28	879	0
Turnip, raw	20	0.3	0.3	0	0
Watermelon, raw	0.3	0.3	4	1,162	0
Yard-long beans, raw	0	0	0	0	0

Taken from Mangles, R.A. et al., "Carotenoid Content of Fruits and Vegetables: An Evaluation of Analytic Data," *Journal of the American Dietetic Association* 93:3 284–296 (1993).

Co-Enzyme Q-10 (Co-Q-10)

The Story of Gina Ferguson

On November 11, 1997, ABC News aired the first in a series of stories on nutrition called "The ABCs of Life." The principal character of that first story was Gina Ferguson. John McKenzie reported:

> Gina Ferguson seemed much too young to be suffering from an enlarged and weakened heart. She was 24 years old, and she was dying.

"I couldn't walk to the bathroom without feeling I had walked a mile," she said. 'Shortness of breath to the point of gasping. The cardiologist they sent me to told me that my life expectancy was very short."

McKenzie: "How short?"

Gina Ferguson: "Ten days."

Doctors already had put her on a variety of powerful medications. Now, running out of ideas, they suggested she try something very different. A little known nutritional supplement. It is called Co-enzyme Q-10.

Dr. Peter Langsjoen, cardiologist: "It doesn't even compare to anything else. Its effects are so clear. They are not subtle. They are dramatic."

What Is Co-Q-10?

So, what is this stuff and why haven't we heard about it?

Co-Q-10 is a vitamin, sort of. It works and acts just like other vitamins, but it has never been recognized as a vitamin officially because of squabbles about the definition of a vitamin. It was first discovered in beef hearts in 1957. In the mid-'60s, it began being used to treat congestive heart failure in Japan. Due largely to the efforts of Dr. Karl Folkers, research began in 1972 to show its benefits in heart disease. That research blossomed in the 1980s, after a method for producing sufficient quantities of it had been mastered in Japan. With increased production, it became one of the top five best-selling drugs in Japan by 1982.

It is also known as "ubiquinone," a conflation of the words "ubiquitous" and "quinone." It is ubiquitous in that it is found in every cell of your body. It is everywhere. A quinone is a biological chemical responsible for creating energy.

Co-Q-10 and the Energy in Our Cells

Co-Q-10 is responsible for the cell's energy in two ways. First, it helps to create at least three of the enzymes the cell uses to create ATP, the fuel created in the mitochondria that is released and burned as energy. Co-Q-10 also creates energy directly, playing a role in the electron and proton transfers as energy passes through the mitochondrial wall and the cell wall. That's right, electrical energy that is released in your cells all the time is controlled in part by this sort-of vitamin that you have never heard of. In addition to that, it acts as an antioxidant.

Where is Co-Q-10 Found?

Ubiquinone can be found in various foods, and it can be taken orally as a supplement. If you want to eat it, about a pound of sardines, two pounds of liver, or two and a half pounds of peanuts will yield about 30 milligrams of Co-Q-10. The dose used in most studies is 100 to 150 milligrams. How hungry are you? For the most part, your body makes its own Co-Q-10. That synthesis is a complex seventeen-stage process that involves eight vitamins (mostly the B vitamins) and several trace minerals. That means a lot of things can go wrong, resulting in not enough Co-Q-10 in your body.

Co-Q-10 and Your Body

To start with, your body starts cutting back on production of Co-Q-10 when you are about twenty years old. This does not make much sense, but that's the way it is. There are three simple reasons why you might not have enough Co-Q-10: you are not getting enough in what you eat, something is blocking your production of it, or your body is burning it up really fast. If you are really not getting enough of it in what you eat, you are probably malnourished and have a major vitamin B deficiency as well. So, let us assume that only applies to cases of serious malnutrition. If you are taking certain medications to block cholesterol formation, like HMG-CoA reductase, that would block Co-Q-10 formation as well. Similar to vitamins A and E, Co-Q-10 is a fat-soluble vitamin and shares certain pathways with cholesterol. This problem can easily be solved by taking more Co-Q-10 into your body with supplements. That's not theory: that is plain, hard fact. *If you are a heart patient taking medication for it, you need a Co-Q-10 supplement.* What does it mean if your body is just burning the stuff up like crazy? That probably means you need to slow down. Excessive bodily consumption of Co-Q-10 can only happen in cases of excessive exertion (running a triathalon every few days), hypermetabolism (going, going, going and drinking lots of coffee, taking pep pills, diet pills, whatever to keep you going), or acute shock states (you have just been hit by a bus). Karl

Folkers believed that what we find as average or "normal" levels of Co-Q-10 are really "suboptimal." We probably all need more than we have. From the number of people I know who are going all the time and never have any energy, he is probably right.

Co-Q-10 and the Heart

Most of the studies involving Co-Q-10 are related to heart and cardiovascular disease. It is low in people who have congestive heart failure. The worse the symptoms are, the lower the Co-Q-10 levels are. When you give these patients Co-Q-10 supplements, they get better 91 percent of the time! What did that say? Ninety-one percent? Cancer treatments are considered really hopeful if they are successful in 25 percent of the cases. Minoxidil, the treatment for baldness, was written up as a miracle cure when it only worked on 33 percent of the men tested. Ninety-one percent is phenomenal!

The Basic Mechanics of the Human Heart

Mechanically speaking, heart failure usually occurs when the muscle responsible for pulling the blood into the heart's main chamber is not doing its job. Pulling the blood into the heart takes a lot more energy than pushing it out, so it is this muscle that is most likely to poop out if the mitochondria cannot make enough energy. It simply runs out of energy, then loses its normally tight muscle tone and begins to relax, causing the heart to enlarge. That then makes it very difficult for it to pull any blood in. Two things happen when the heart is not pumping enough blood: blood pressure rises (trying to compensate for the broken pump), and the heart muscle starts trying to work really hard. Your heart may start beating faster. If your heart begins beating faster and faster and yet it does not sense any blood going through it, there is a distinct possibility that your heart might have an electrical blowout called a myocardial infarction (heart attack). Co-Q-10 makes the heart pump more blood with each beat, the heart rate slows down, the size of the heart muscle goes down, no more chest pains, and no more fatigue. Twenty different studies and over three hundred papers all agree on the effectiveness and safety of Co-Q-10. It reduces the risk of LDL cholesterol, the cause of atherosclerosis, and oxidation as well.

Co-Q-10 Can Be Used with Other Cardiovascular-Disease Drugs

Co-Q-10 can be used in conjunction with any of the drugs usually used to treat cardiovascular disease and it will not conflict with them. Langsjoen found that more than half of his patients with high blood pressure could stop taking one or more of their medicines within four months after starting Co-Q-10. He also found that of all 424 cardiovascular patients, 43 percent were able to drop one to three of their medications with ubiquinone therapy. Some patients, the ones who started treatments at the first sign of a problem, were able to regain normal heart function and size with Co-Q-10 alone. Consult your physician about adding Co-Q-10 to your treatment program.

The Success of Co-Q-10 in Treating the Human Heart

Because of the success of ubiquinone in treating the heart, research is only beginning to understand the roles it plays in other diseases. The fact that it is an antioxidant that gradually diminishes as we grow older automatically relates it to aging and the degenerative diseases involved in that process. We just need to know details. If Co-Q-10 is essential for giving energy (translate that "life") to every cell of the body, we would expect that it will be involved in other diseases, too.

Co-Q-10 and Periodontal Disease

A dental researcher serving in the Air Force found that patients with periodontal disease also had low Co-Q-10 levels. Dentists say that half of the patients they see have some degree of gum disease, and this is the leading cause of tooth loss in those over sixty years of age. Simple supplementation with Co-Q-10 reversed this condition. No doubt this was due to the antioxidant effect of Co-Q-10 reversing oxidative degeneration of the tissue.

Co-Q-10 in Mice Slowed the Aging Process

Researchers at UCLA showed that mice given supplements of Co-Q-10 entered old age looking younger, with healthier fur and with more energy. This would indicate that its antioxidant effects slowed the aging process and might extend life.

Co-Q-10 Also Boosts the Immune System

The immune system is boosted also. Aging can lower the number of antibodies to about one third of the number found in young, healthy people. Co-Q-10 given to the elderly stimulates production of antibodies by two and a half times and can restore the immune system to about 80 percent of its original potency. It has also been noted that end-stage AIDS patients are remarkably deficient of Co-Q-10.

Co-Q-10 and Chemotherapy

There has not been much to associate Co-Q-10 with cancer, but boosting of the immune system is a start. It has also been found that the toxicity of the chemotherapy drug Adriamycin can be reduced by Co-Q-10. This has a significant effect on the ability of people to survive chemotherapy.

Co-Q-10 and Parkinson's Disease

Recent studies, in August 1997 and February 1998, have linked ubiquinone with Parkinson's disease. The first found that Co-Q-10 levels were low in untreated Parkinson's patients and that there were correspondingly low levels of complexes I and II/III, the enzymes that Co-Q-10 controls. The second study found that supplementation was able to reduce the loss of dopamine that occurs in Parkinson's disease. Dopamine is a hormone precursor that is essential for transmitting nerve signals, especially those that affect motor control and mood.

Co-Q-10 and the Prevention of Oxidative Damage in the Human Brain

A Polish paper recently showed that Co-Q-10 supplements can prevent oxidative damage in the brain, such as lesions and neurological damage, that can come from spasms of the blood vessels in the brain. This type of damage is caused by free radical damage to fats in the blood plasma and leads to memory loss, stroke, or cancer. Co-Q-10 can reduce the risk of all of these by controlling oxidative damage.

So, Why Don't Americans Know About Co-Q-10?

As to why you probably have not heard of it before, Co-Q-10 is not patentable. Most medicines are developed by a single company that advertises its product and educates both doctors and the public about the benefits of that product, knowing that it is the only company that will reap the benefits in terms of sales. No one company can do that with Co-Q-10, because they can't shut out the competition. As you might guess, advertising and education is expensive and without the guarantee of returns, no company will take on the burden of promotion.

What Happened to Gina?

By the way, remember Gina Ferguson, who had ten days to live? A month after she began taking Co-Q-10, her heart was measurably improved. "The end result is that I'm still here. I can still be a mother to my child and I can still be a wife. Co-enzyme Q-10, for me, is my lifeline."

Co-Q-10 Benefits Include . . . Co-enzyme Q-10 (Co-Q-10) is also known as ubiquinone. It has been used in Japan since the 1970s as a treatment for various heart and circulatory problems, becoming one of the top five best-selling drugs in the country by 1982.

Among its many benefits are: 1) generation of energy to every cell in the body; 2) prevention and treatment of a wide variety of cardiovascular diseases, including congestive heart failure, angina pectoris, cardiac arrhythmias, high blood pressure, and atherosclerosis; 3) prevention and treatment of cancer of the breast, lung, colon, prostate, and other types of cancer; 4) treatment of several types of muscular dystrophy; 5) treatment of periodontal disease; 6) protection against cellular damage of excessive free radical activity; and 7) slowing of various aspects of the aging process, leading to the extension of mean lifespan in animal studies.

Co-Q-10 Dosages: The recommended dosage in most of the studies is 90 to 150 milligrams, but many people simply do not respond at this dosage. Chances are that, if you are not responding to lower doses, the product you are taking is not being sufficiently absorbed by your body. The issue of bioavailability is important for all supplements: Does your body actually get to use all of the nutrient that is on the label? In many cases, the nutrient bonds to other chemicals in the formula or is not even dissolved in the digestive tract. Just because they put it in the pill does not mean the pill gets it to your body. Dr. Stephan Sinatra, in his *Heart Sense* newsletter, says, "You may be receiving far less strength than the label indicates and your less than energetic lifestyle may bear witness to that." Co-Q-10 seems to be absorbed better in the presence of brewer's yeast or RNA/DNA. Also, it is best taken in an oil base. I recommend a dosage range of 100 to 200 mg.

DHEA

DHEA is an abbreviation for *dehydroepiandrosterone*. Careful trying to pronounce it: You could hurt yourself. We'll just stick with the letters DHEA. So what is this stuff?

What Is DHEA and What Does It Do?

In a lot of ways, it is like melatonin (see pages 193–204). It is a hormone, only recently discovered, that starts diminishing after you reach a certain age, so it is associated with the aging process. It affects brain function and slows memory loss. Its causes deeper sleep. As an antioxidant, it can reduce the risk of cardiovascular disease and reduce the risk of some cancers. In these ways, it is much like melatonin.

But the differences between melatonin and DHEA are what make it important. First, it is produced by the adrenal gland, the same gland that makes adrenaline (the excitement hormone). Remember that we said this is one of the glands controlled by the pineal gland through melatonin. Second, though melatonin is gender-blind, DHEA works best in men. Next, it shuts off production a little sooner, between the ages of thirty and forty, so that by the time you are between fifty and seventy years old, you have only about 20 percent of the amount of DHEA you had as a young adult. Also, we haven't learned as much yet about DHEA as we have about melatonin. Research takes time. Most of the studies are still being done on mice. The biggest difference is that, while melatonin is pretty safe, DHEA can have some side effects that you really do not want. We will talk about those in detail later. First, let's see what DHEA can do for us.

DHEA Stimulates!

The key word for understanding DHEA is *stimulate*! While melatonin balances, DHEA excites! It stimulates the brain; it stimulates the immune system; it stimulates the muscles to promote more lean muscle mass and less fat; it stimulates the sex hormones estrogen and testosterone; it even stimulates the pancreas to produce more insulin. Before we get overstimulated here, let's slow down and look at details.

DHEA Linked to Increasing or Preserving Muscle Mass

Many of the antiaging effects of DHEA are linked to its ability to increase or preserve muscle mass. On the simplest level, it reduces "middle-age spread" by cutting back the body fat and promoting lean muscle mass. Most of us who have passed thirty have found we just cannot eat as much pizza as we used to and we have seen our waistbands stretch into numbers are embarrassed to admit. The normal reduction in DHEA may be the reason our metabolism changes about that time. Geoffry Cowley, who wrote an article for *Newsweek* on DHEA, noticed that he personally, after thirty days of DHEA supplements and weight training, gained six pounds of muscle and dropped his body fat from 7 percent to 5.4 percent in just one month. That observation is hardly scientific, but it makes the point. Reduction of excess fat can have tremendous benefits of all kinds. It reduces the risk of heart problems and onset diabetes. It would increase our energy levels and improve our mood. It would do wonders for our self-image if we could just control our body shape.

There is also a connection between muscle wasting and chronic heart failure. The National Heart and Lung Institute in London recently found that the same connection extended to DHEA levels. Lower DHEA levels were directly associated with both loss in muscle mass and the severity of chronic heart failure, but their study went even further. In trying to figure out all the mechanics involved, they also found that heart failure and muscle wasting had to do with the change from anabolic to catabolic metabolism. Say what? There was a change from the kind of metabolism where food is changed into body-building tissue (anabolic), which is governed by DHEA, to a metabolism where the body is eating away at its own tissue for energy (catabolic), which is ruled by cortisol, another product of the adrenal gland. The drop in DHEA actually changes the way your body gets its energy so that it goes from building itself up with food to tearing itself down by "eating itself." This doesn't just happen overnight. It is long process that progresses slowly and is measured as a ratio of cortisol to DHEA. The more DHEA, the less wasting; the more cortisol, the more the body is consuming itself instead of food. So, what does it do with the food? It begins storing it as fat, of course. Now back up and read the paragraph before this. It might start making sense.

Muscle Mass and DHEA Levels

Let's carry this process out to its logical conclusion. A study was made of people age 90 to 106 in an Italian community to see why some functioned better than others in old age. They found that the two most significant factors in old people maintaining physical independence were muscle mass and high DHEA levels.[18] The people who had severe age-related impairments were poorly educated, institutionalized, had sensory impairment (blindness, deafness, etc.), atrophied muscles, and lower DHEA levels. *Science* magazine reported in the same month that loss of muscle mass leading to frailty is the leading cause of death in the oldest part of the population and that this loss is related to the decline in hormone activity. All together, those who maintained an active mind and strong muscles survived better in old age. Higher DHEA is related to both of those effects. Those who had higher DHEA levels still had metabolisms geared toward building, but those who had lost DHEA had begun the process of tearing down their own vital tissues in order to survive.

DHEA and Diabetes

Increased body fat is a major problem for diabetics because it wreaks havoc with both their blood sugar and their resistance to insulin, but DHEA has provided new avenues of research into helping control this disease. First, it reduces body fat. Researchers at Washington University (Jan. 1998) gave DHEA to diabetic rats and found that they lost 25 percent of their body fat without any changes in muscle mass or the amount of food they ate! Both that study and another at the University of Naples, Italy, (October 1997) found that DHEA levels in the blood determine the amount of insulin resistance. After measuring insulin effectiveness, testosterone, and DHEA levels in seventy-five people ages

21 to 106, they found that the increase in insulin resistance that had previously been associated with age was really dependent on DHEA levels. So, DHEA's work in reducing fat and increasing muscle is extremely important in avoiding the onset of diabetes and in controlling its progress. In fact, DHEA has even been found to reverse Type II diabetes,[19] the type found in overweight, middle-aged men and women.

DHEA Helps in Fighting Spikes in Blood Sugar Levels

In addition to the benefits listed above, DHEA has antioxidant properties that we are just beginning to understand. In relation to diabetes, DHEA, given to rats three hours before a shot of pure dextrose (sugar), was able to significantly reduce the amount of lipid peroxidation and free radical damage normally associated with surges of high blood sugar found in the brain, liver, and kidneys. The diabetic has to fight these spikes in his blood sugar with every meal and small amounts of tissue damaged with each episode add up in the long run, leading to blindness, impotence, kidney failure, and circulatory problems that can result in amputation. If DHEA levels can be maintained, that free radical damage can be controlled. At the same time, DHEA increases the person's sensitivity to insulin so that the spikes of blood sugar are not as high.

DHEA Linked with Raising Glutathione Levels

Another important role for DHEA in relation to antioxidants was just reported in March 1998. E. L. White and researchers at the Southern Research Institute in Birmingham, Alabama, were looking for chemicals they could use in chemotherapy that would raise glutathione levels without making the patient sick. If you remember, glutathione is the enzyme most responsible for stopping lipid peroxidation in cells, and because of this, it is strongly related to controlling the growth of cancers. Among the seven chemicals they found acceptable for further research was DHEA. By boosting glutathione production and preventing lipid peroxidation (rancidity), DHEA takes us a long way in our battle against one of the most dangerous aspects of oxidative stress.

The Role of DHEA in Battling Cancer

The role of DHEA in battling cancer may be remarkable. It both boosts the immune system and reduces Reactive Oxygen Species (ROS) damage. When given to rats with virus-induced leukemia, DHEA dramatically reduced free radical activity and, at the same time, boosted the production of IL-2, a cancer-fighting immune stimulator.[20] Another study also found DHEA to bring back normal production of IL-10, an immune regulator, which normally disappears with aging, then overresponds when needed, attacking healthy cells. The bottom line is that the major effects of infecting these rats with leukemia were undone by the benefits of DHEA.

Burn Damage and DHEA

Burn damage is one of the most complicated medical problems because the healing process is slow and goes through several stages, each of which has its own complications. There is also a danger to the surrounding tissues, which have reduced blood flow and greater exposure to infection. Free radicals stir up trouble at every turn in this process. DHEA helps burns heal much faster and better. Barbara A. Araneo of the University of Utah Medical School also cites the immune-stimulating function of DHEA as an important factor in healing burns.

DHEA Benefits for Women as Well as Men

We had said that men respond better to DHEA than women, but there are some benefits that are especially for women. A feminine benefit from DHEA is that, when given to postmenopausal women as a vaginal cream, their vaginas were restored to the condition of a mature woman and, at the same time, bone formation was stimulated. This means that it should be considered as a treatment for osteoporosis.

What Are the Downsides of DHEA?

With all that going for it, you might wonder why it's not showing up on every other television commercial as a miracle aging cure.

There are two reasons. First, there have not been enough long-term studies in humans to know what would happen if someone took supplements for thirty years. Second, the side effects can be really serious. If you start giving DHEA to postmenopausal women (who have low estrogen levels), it may increase their risk of breast cancer. Because DHEA stimulates both estrogen and testosterone, it could actually cause some types of cancer to spread like crazy. The same hormones can stimulate facial hair on women and breast growth in men. There may also be a threat of liver damage.

Until we know more about how the hormone works, it must be used with caution. Don't start using it without a blood test to determine your current blood levels of DHEA and related hormones. That means you will have to consult with a doctor about it, but make sure that doctor is knowledgeable about the latest advances in hormone therapy. Most doctors are totally in the dark on this subject and think it is nonsense. A few would like to treat everyone for everything with DHEA. Avoid both extremes and find a responsible endocrinologist to help you determine the best course for you. If you are under thirty years old, you do not need to think about it. Anyone who has a family history of breast, ovary, or prostate cancer probably should not use it except under a doctor's strict supervision.

DHEA Supplementation

Honestly, some of the data looks great, and some does not. One study said that DHEA had no effect on weight loss, but they studied obese teenagers whose DHEA level are still high normally. Their obesity had nothing to do with the metabolism change that we have been talking about. Another study could not detect any measurable difference in cognitive ability. But in August 1997, a study with rats was the first to show that supplementation "completely reversed" the age-related reduction of hormones, not only DHEA but all the essential hormones involved along the hypothalamus/pituitary/adrenal axis. That leads us to believe that supplementation will work; we just have to find the right ways to use it. My suggested dosage is 25 to 50 mg for women and 50 to 100 mg for men.

Mexican Yams Do Not Raise Your Blood DHEA Levels

There is a rumor out there that you can increase your DHEA by taking its precursors, which are extracted from Mexican yams or wild yams. Mexican yams do not raise your blood DHEA levels. Stick with real DHEA from a top-quality manufacturer who guarantees standardized dosages. There is no telling what kind of binders or contaminants might be in products of lesser quality. DHEA blood levels, like melatonin, can also be preserved, or at least the decline is slowed, by reducing calorie intake.[21]

Enzymes

Free Radical Scavenging Systems

Another weapon your body has for fighting free radicals is its enzyme systems. Enzymes are chemical compounds that the body creates to act as catalysts in various kinds of chemical reactions that need to take place. The enzymes we will be talking about are created at the cellular level and facilitate chemical reactions at that level. Specifically, there are five enzymes that fight oxidation caused by hydrogen peroxide, two of which work together. They are superoxide dismutase, catalase, glutathione peroxidase, glutathione reductase, and glutathione transferase.

Superoxide Dismutase

Superoxide dismutase (SOD) is the enzyme that neutralizes the superoxide radical. It is a chain-breaking antioxidant, important because it can stop a chain reaction of free radical damage even while it is occurring. The SOD takes apart superoxide and creates hydrogen peroxide and oxygen. Hydrogen peroxide is much weaker than superoxide, but still dangerous. Superoxide dismutase requires the enzyme catalase then to remove the hydrogen peroxide molecules. Catalase is abundant in our body's red blood cells and helps to remove hydrogen peroxide from our system, from our tissues. This prevents formation of the more toxic free radicals. Glutathione teams up with selenium to combat peroxides, such as hydrogen peroxide.

The end result of the work of SOD is that the superoxide is gone, but hydrogen peroxide is left as a by-product. To deal with that problem, other enzymes immediately come into play.

Catalase

Catalase is abundant in our body's red blood cells and helps to remove hydrogen peroxide from our system, from our tissues. This prevents formation of the more toxic free radicals. Methionine supplementation has been shown to result in higher catalase and peroxidase enzyme activities.

Catalase, simply put, is an enzyme that converts hydrogen peroxide to water. It causes a reaction that combines two molecules of H_2O_2 to make two molecules of H_2O and one of O_2, (oxygen). Much of the hydrogen peroxide metabolized by catalase is produced by the action of SOD in neutralizing superoxide. Where SOD finishes, catalase takes over and turns the toxic hydrogen peroxide into water and oxygen. The limitation of catalase is that it will not metabolize cellular lipid peroxides, which are formed by free radicals. What does this mean? That is, it will not break down the peroxide in the cell wall or attached to other fatty acids in the cell. It only attacks the peroxide that is free floating in the water-soluble parts of the cell. This is important in that it stops the hydrogen peroxide that might affect the mitochondria and DNA of the cell. To get to the lipid peroxides, we must turn to glutathione peroxidase.

Gluthathione Peroxidase

Glutathione peroxidase also converts hydrogen peroxide to water, but it tends to metabolize hydrogen peroxide missed by catalase. In other words, it functions a bit like your certified public accountant in correcting and cleaning up missed mathematical errors in any Internal Revenue Service forms you are working on. The mistakes you did not catch, your CPA will soon correct; the hydrogen peroxide that catalase missed the first time will be cleaned up and removed by glutathione peroxidase. Glutathione peroxidase has the ability to remove the peroxide formed in membrane fatty acids. This metabolism of membrane lipid peroxide allows for the repair of cell membranes. So, between these two enzymes, all of the hydrogen peroxide that might appear in a cell can be defeated before it does serious damage. Back to the CPA-IRS tax forms analogy: between your review and that of your CPA, all of your mathematical errors will have been found and corrected prior to submission of any paperwork to our dear IRS. The trace mineral selenium is essential for the activity of glutathione peroxidase. Those who are selenium deficient cannot synthesize glutathione peroxidase and thereby are susceptible to free radical activity, especially from hydrogen peroxide.

Glutathione Reductase

Additionally, glutathione peroxidase is a complex enzyme requiring adequate supplies of glutathione for its activity. When glutathione and glutathione peroxidase get together to neutralize some free radicals, the glutathione ends up in its disulfide form, called GSSG. This must be reduced back to glutathione by the activity of glutathione reductase, the third enzyme we identified. It does not fight free radicals itself, but it turns GSSG back into glutathione so that glutathione peroxidase can do its job.

Glutathione is a tripeptide (a simple protein) consisting of three amino acids and found in almost every human cell. Glutathione reductase is responsible for transforming the altered peptide back to a form usable by glutathione peroxidase.

(Take a Breather . . .)

Confused yet? Much of this information is fairly complex. You may wish to simply skim through this enzyme section to get a general idea of what is going on inside your body, but know that this information is here if you need it for reference purposes. Many times we hear or read new terminology and the underlying concepts don't really hit us until we are able to get a more complete understanding of how the whole process works.

Glutathione Transferase

Glutathione transferase is another enzyme that is a potent lipid peroxide scavenger. It serves both as a backup and a complementary system to glutathione peroxidase. Experimentation is currently being done to see if direct supplementation of this enzyme can increase immune reactions in AIDS patients.

What happens when there is not enough glutathione or selenium for the enzymes to do their job? If hydrogen peroxide is not completely converted to water, the hydroxyl radical, a very toxic free radical cellular component, is formed. This conversion of hydrogen peroxide to hydroxyl radicals is enhanced in the presence of iron or other metals. Intercellular hemorrhage can release iron from the red blood cells, which acts as a catalyst to convert hydrogen peroxide to the toxic hydroxyl radical. So, if the enzyme system fails, an opposite set of reactions occurs to perpetuate more free radical damage in the cell.

The hydroxyl radicals are the most toxic of the free radicals. There is no specific enzymatic defense against it. The hydroxyl radical causes changes in the structure of the cell membrane and alters its permeability, leaking calcium into the cell and ultimately leading to the cell's self-destruction.

A free radical of any type can interact with the fatty acids in the cell membrane, producing lipid peroxides. The hydroxyl radical and other free radicals steal an electron from the fatty acids and, after undergoing molecular rearrangement, they themselves become free radicals. This continued peroxidation of the membrane further weakens the membrane. Along with glutathione peroxidase, vitamin E and other free radical scavengers interact with the peroxidative processes of the lipids in the cell membrane and neutralize them.

Free radicals are not limited to oxygen compounds. Any molecule that has an extra electron in its outer orbit is by definition a free radical. A drug can become a free radical during its metabolism. A "free radical drug" can initiate the same lipid peroxidation of the cell membrane and DNA damage within the cell as an oxygen radical.

Factors That Regulate the Ability to Scavenge Free Radicals

Normally, enzyme free radical–scavenging activity occurs in every cell, but there are specific factors that may enhance or subdue this activity. The first of these factors to consider is the *total burden* of free radicals the body confronts. General Custer's troops lost the battle at Little Big Horn for a simple reason: too many Indians. In the same way, the limited number of antioxidants in your body can be overrun by too many oxidants. Free radicals are generated continuously, so it is essential to provide the cells with the best possible conditions for dealing with them. For each cellular component there is a specific concentration that must be reached before cellular damage occurs. Given the right circumstances, the activity of free radical–scavenging enzymes maintain free radical concentrations below this minimum toxic concentration (MTC). The safety margin between free radical concentration and the MTC is wide, but that safety margin decreases as the total free radical burden increases. The more oxidation occurring in a cell, the less efficiently the body is able to control it.

Genetic Regulation

Genetic regulation is another factor that controls both the absolute quantity and the efficiency of each free radical–scavenging enzyme. Each individual has a different capacity and rate of scavenging free radicals. Patients with genetically low absolute concentrations of free radical–scavenging enzymes are more susceptible to free radical damage at the cellular level. Consequently, they are more susceptible to free radical induced or mediated disease. This is one reason why longevity, certain diseases, and a specific rate of aging can be seen in families. Often it is equally evident that one family member ages more rapidly or has more disease and breaks the pattern because of tobacco and/or alcohol use. In such a case, that individual's ability to deal with oxidation was the same as the other family members, but his or her intake of oxidants and antioxidant inhibitors was greater.

Nutritional Status

Nutritional status can decrease free radical–enzyme scavenging activity. Your body needs what it needs. You can't expect to be deficient in some vitamin or mineral and not be affected by it. Marginal vitamin deficiencies, particularly of vitamins C and E, can decrease the cell's ability to scavenge free radicals. Even cellular depletion of certain trace elements leads to decreased free radical–enzyme scavenging activity. Conversely, adequate amounts of these elements lead to efficient antioxidant functioning. These trace elements are essential cofactors for the synthesis and proper functioning of the free radical–scavenging enzymes. We have already mentioned selenium as a cofactor necessary for the production of glutathione peroxidase. Organic iron is needed for catalase to do its job. Inappropriate nutrition can lead to marginal deficiencies in some of the cofactors necessary for maximum free radical–scavenging activity. But even marginal deficiencies can lead to devastating effects if oxidation is not controlled.

Drug Therapy

Drug therapy effects enzymatic antioxidant systems in two ways. First, drugs, prescription or otherwise, can produce marginal deficiencies of trace elements by depleting cellular trace element concentrations. Also, drug metabolism can increase the total burden of free radicals. Increases in the total burden of free radicals often occur during drug administration. Most drugs are intended to shock the system into fighting certain symptoms, but this shock tends to pull trace elements away from their normal function and increase oxidation. Free radicals then are produced by almost all drugs as they are metabolized into less toxic compounds. For example, Adriamycin is an anticancer drug that is highly toxic to the heart because of the oxidative stress it creates. But Dr. Horie has found that the antioxidant properties of aged garlic extract nullifies its threat to the heart without interfering with its intended cancer-fighting properties. Therefore, drug metabolism places an excessive free radical load on the capacity of an individual's system of free radical–scavenging enzymes and depletes its ability to deal with that load.

Environmental Factors

Environmental factors can also increase the total burden of free radicals. Pollution, secondhand smoke, emotional stress, and many other factors may increase cellular oxidation. Any sudden excessive increase in the total burden of free radicals that is secondary to therapeutic, dietary, or environmental factors can lead to free radical cell membrane damage. Radiation, in the form of electromagnetic fields, is unavoidable in our culture ruled by computers, microwaves, and high-tension power lines. Even the radiation from sunlight increases oxidation. Pesticides and other contaminants in our food sources and water significantly affect the diseases prevalent here as compared to countries with simpler farming methods. Many of these environmental factors can be controlled if we are aware and take appropriate measures, like drinking purified water. Other factors cannot be controlled, and the oxidation they cause must be accounted for in our supplementation.

All of the factors listed above can alter the efficiency of the free radical–scavenging systems. Regardless of the underlying cause, when the minimum toxic concentration (MTC) is exceeded, cellular damage occurs and the patient will ultimately exhibit clinical symptoms of the disease process. Which disease shows up will be determined by which enzyme systems within which organs have failed and where the toxic concentration is. This means it is absolutely necessary to see to it that the system has everything it needs to function properly.

These enzyme scavenging systems are designed as a fail-safe system to prevent the formation of hydroxyl radicals. Since there is no enzyme to scavenge the hydroxyl radical, failure of the free radical–scavenging system places more burden on other systems to rid the body of this toxin. The success of the enzyme system is dependent on a number of factors, including the presence of adequate amounts of selenium, glutathione, and glutathione reductase. When these factors are absent in a given patient, the probability that the patient will develop free radical–mediated disease increases significantly.

Exercise May Be a Double-Edged Sword: As Dr. Arnold J. Susser states, "[e]xercise may be a two-edged sword. Don't think that exercise alone is sufficient to protect you from the age-afflicting ravages of free radicals. As a matter of fact, a 1993 article in a magazine on sports exercise reported that exercise can actually increase the level of free radicals in the system."[1]

Dr. Cooper, the aerobic exercise guru, has announced the same findings. In fact, Susser continues, "[a]ging may cause not only an overall elevation of antioxidant enzyme activities, but also a fiber-specific adaptation of GSH system (in skeletal muscle). Exercise training, although increasing selective antioxidant enzymes in the young, does not offer additional protection against oxidative stress in the senescent muscle. Therefore, exercise, to be maximally effective in combating aging, must be supplemented by super antioxidants!"[2]

Garlic

Dr. Benjamin Lau, M.D., Ph.D.'s "GARLIC" acronym to summarize its major health benefits:

G =   good for many things
A =   antioxidant effects
R =   restoration of memory
L =   life extension
I =   immune modulation
C =   cancer prevention.[22]

Garlic and Its Importance

On occasion, patients will ask me: "If I could only take one supplement, what should it be?" The question may come because they are concerned about the cost of a multitude of vitamins and minerals. Or it may simply be intended to clarify priorities in what needs to be taken. Inevitably, no matter what their condition is, my answer is *garlic*!

Garlic's Healing Qualities Known Throughout History

Garlic is one of the oldest medical remedies known to man and used in almost all cultures throughout history. The earliest reference to garlic as a medication is in the Ebers Papyrus from sixteenth century B.C.E. Egypt, which lists twenty-two remedies using garlic. The builders of the Pyramids were paid in the valuable commodities of onions and garlic, and preserved garlic was found in King Tut's tomb. In the Greek world, Homer, Aristotle, and Hippocrates all cited garlic's healing qualities, and it is said that ancient Olympic athletes would chew a clove of garlic before competing. The East Indians used it for treating wounds. The Chinese have used onion tea for centuries to relieve cholera and dysentery. The voyages of the Vikings and Phoenicians were always well stocked with garlic. After the Crusaders brought garlic to France, it became so popular as a curative agent that King Henry IV ate a clove of raw garlic every morning. Garlic was also a key ingredient in the famous Four Thieves' vinegar, used to fight the plague in Marseilles in the 1770s. More recently, Louis Pasteur recognized garlic's antibacterial properties, and Albert Schweitzer gave out garlic to treat dysentery when his medical supplies ran out. Physicians have long reported the healing powers of garlic. Improvements in asthma, tuberculosis, bronchitis, stomach ulcers, athletes' foot, leg ulcers, the respiratory tract, lungs, and other body systems were documented.

What Are Garlic's Positive Health Effects?

Garlic has the following positive health effects:

1. acts as a super antioxidant,
2. lowers blood pressure,
3. boosts the immune system,
4. balances blood sugar,
5. prevents heart disease,
6. assists in fat metabolism,
7. relieves intermittent claudication, and,
8. aids in cancer prevention.

Why Is Garlic Considered a Powerful Antioxidant?

The reason garlic is such a powerful antioxidant is because it is loaded with most of the phytonutrients we consider to be the super antioxidants. It contains manganese, selenium, germanium, vitamin A, vitamin C, and zinc.

Garlic and Lowering Your Blood Pressure

Garlic is known to be one of the most effective agents for lowering blood pressure. It has been found to lower both diastolic and systolic blood pressure.

Garlic and Boosting Your Immune System

Garlic has long been known to be an important stimulator of the body's defense system. Garlic's sulfur compounds enhance the function of the white blood cells. These white blood cells function most efficiently when the body is supplied with appropriate antioxidant nutrients, especially the sulfur compounds. Selenium and germanium are potent sulfur-containing antioxidants found in garlic. The immune system's T-helper cells are also stimulated. A study by Dr. Tariq Abdullah showed that the natural killer cells of patients who ate raw garlic killed 139 percent more tumor cells in laboratory cultures. Those who used kyolic capsules killed 159 percent more!

Garlic Is Known to Have Antiviral, Antibacterial, and Antifungal Effects

Garlic is also known to have positive, direct antiviral, antibacterial, and antifungal effects. It has been used at Hunan Medical College in China to treat a deadly form of meningitis caused by the *Cryptococcus neoformans* microbe. Dr. Benjamin Lau also reports his use of garlic to aid patients with chronic fatigue (associated with the Epstein-Barr virus), the cytomegalovirus, the Coxsackie virus, and the herpes virus. A study at Tufts University showed that garlic was effective against *Entamoeba histolytica*, which causes amebic dysentery. Additionally, garlic removes toxic heavy metals as a chelator. These heavy metals, such as mercury and lead, impair immune function.

Garlic and Balancing Your Blood Sugar Levels

Garlic has been shown in many studies to lower blood sugar levels. If you have a tendency toward hypoglycemia and want to take advantage of garlic's other benefits without lowering blood sugar further, use aged garlic extract (Kyolic garlic). It will not dangerously lower your blood sugar. Instead, it will stabilize your sugar, preventing wide fluctuations. Raw garlic does lower blood sugar and could be potentially dangerous to the hypoglycemic.

Garlic and the Prevention of Heart Disease

The key to heart health is encouraging the "good" HDL (high-density lipoprotein) cholesterol and limiting the "bad" LDL (low-density lipoprotein) cholesterol. Actually, LDL itself is not so bad, but it becomes dangerous when it is oxidized by free radicals inside a blood vessel. When that happens, it is attacked by the white blood cells, which become engorged and are then deposited on the arterial wall as plaque This leads to thickening of the arterial wall, narrowing of the passageway, and eventually blockage. HDL, on the other hand, being denser and heavier, is not likely to attach itself to the arterial wall. Instead, it actually picks up LDL, pulling it away from the blood vessel, and transporting it to the liver, where it can be broken down and excreted.

At the fourth International Congress of Phytotherapy in Munich, Germany, in 1992, Dr. Jorg GruenWald concluded that garlic protects the heart and arteries in two ways: 1) "Garlic reduces the free radicals that cause damage to cholesterol. Undamaged LDL cholesterol is harmless, but in its oxidized form is extremely dangerous to the arterial walls resulting in arteriosclerosis. Therefore, by inhibiting the oxidative stress from free radicals on LDL cholesterol, this process of arteriosclerosis can be inhibited"; and 2) "Garlic also inhibits the infiltration of damaged fats and cholesterol through the wall of the arteries." Further, "if cholesterol is so overabundant at one site that it tries to push its way through an arterial wall, or a damaged LDL cholesterol molecule tries to damage an artery, garlic will inhibit this process." Dr. Lau's studies in 1987 revealed much the same information, showing that garlic reduced the levels of LDL cholesterol while increasing the levels of HDL cholesterol, which are likely to pick LDL off the arterial wall.

Garlic Supplements Are Licensed as Drugs Against Arteriosclerosis in Germany

This two-level protection is impressive. Add to it garlic's ability to lower serum cholesterol, triglycerides, and blood pressure, and its ability to reduce platelet aggregation and premature clotting, and we can understand why garlic is the single most important food for protecting the heart and arteries. It should be noted that garlic supplements are licensed as drugs against arteriosclerosis in Germany.

More Studies Confirming Garlic's Benefits in Treating Heart Patients

A study in India took 432 patients who had already had a heart attack and gave half of them daily garlic supplements. At the end of three years, those who took the garlic had fewer additional heart attacks, lower blood pressure, and lower serum cholesterol. Also, twice as many people in the control group died during the study as in the group who took garlic. The results were attributed to the garlic dissolving atherosclerotic blockages in the coronary arteries. Another study, at a heart disease center in Heidelberg, indicated that regular garlic intake decreased the stiffness of the aorta, which normally shows increasing stiffness with age.

Garlic and the Prevention of Heart Attacks and Strokes

As if that were not enough, garlic contains a compound called ajoene, which is as potent as aspirin in preventing red blood cells from clumping together. At the same time, other components in garlic lengthen clotting time and others dissolve clots. Garlic makes every aspect of blood flow and coagulation work properly, and all three of these actions have a positive effect in prevention of heart attacks and strokes.

Garlic's Assistance in Metabolizing Fat

Fat enters our blood from three sources: 1) food intake, 2) endogenous lipogenesis (the fat made by our body), and 3) failure of the body to break down fat and eliminate it. The amount of fat we take in is totally within our control if we are aware of the fat content of the foods we eat. Younger, active people usually burn the fat they take in, but as a person gets older and more sedentary, the fat tends to go straight from the lips to the hips. As to the second and third sources of fat, our body regulates these things without consulting our ideal weight chart and body sculpting goals. What we can do is to give our body what it needs to produce less fat and metabolize it efficiently. Alcohol, for example, tends to increase blood and tissue lipids by sparking endogenous lipogenesis and interfering with the breakdown of dietary fats. Garlic, on the other hand, assists in metabolizing fat in at least three ways.

According to Dr. Benjamin Lau, "garlic has been shown to either inhibit or reduce endogenous lipogenesis . . . to increase breakdown of lipids and to enhance elimination of the breakdown byproducts through the intestinal tract . . . [and] garlic has been shown to move lipids from the tissue depot to the blood circulation and subsequently excreted from the body."[23] Garlic works so well, in fact, that one researcher fed rats a high-fat diet, gave them alcohol, mixed it with garlic oil, and the rats showed *no increase* in blood or tissue lipids.

Garlic and the Relief of Intermittent Claudication

Some people find that they begin having pain or weakness in their legs when they walk for a while, but the symptoms stop when they stop walking. This is called intermittent claudication and it occurs because of poor blood circulation in the legs. Garlic is extremely effective in improving circulation in the peripheral vasculature where blood flow may be impeded because of clogged arteries. In one study, over thirty patients were studied for a three-month period wherein their diet was supplemented with garlic. Each suffered from claudication. Each improved their walking distance before symptoms of claudication occurred. In addition, blood pressure, cholesterol, and spontaneous clotting decreased dramatically, all attributed to garlic supplementation.

Garlic and the Prevention of Cancer

Many laboratory experiments have shown that garlic is a powerful inhibitor of cancer. Both fresh garlic and aged garlic extract have shown this benefit. One of the key reasons for this is the complex of antioxidants, like selenium and bioflavonoids, contained in garlic.

Kyolic Garlic Extract Inhibited Aflatoxin from Binding to DNA

Aflatoxin is strongly linked with liver and other forms of cancer. It is produced by the *Aspergillus* mold, which contaminates peanuts, rice, corn, beans, and many other foods, and is strongly linked with liver and other forms of cancer. Aflatoxin is not a carcinogen in its natural form but becomes cancer-causing when it is oxidized into its "epoxid form" in our bodies. The epoxid form binds to DNA and RNA, affecting the replication of the cell and leading to mutation. Dr. Lau's studies determined that "[K]yolic garlic extract inhibited aflatoxin from binding to DNA. Further, it also inhibited the oxidation of aflatoxin to the epoxid form and additionally increased the levels of glutathione conjugates which are important in the whole antioxidant mechanism against cancer."[24]

M. D. Anderson Hospital Doctors Shocked by Garlic Compound's Cancer Protection

In one study at M. D. Anderson Hospital, Dr. Michael Wargovich found that mice given both diallyl sulfide (a component of garlic) and a colon-specific carcinogen developed 75 percent fewer tumors. But when the same procedure was used with a carcinogen that affects the esophagus, Dr. Wargovich remarked, "[w]e were shocked at the end of that experiment. Even though the garlic-treated animals were exposed to one of the most potent carcinogens around, *not one got cancer*. We believe diallyl sulfide triggers the liver to detoxify carcinogens."

Other Research Also Supportive of Garlic's Many Benefits

Other population and laboratory studies lead to similar conclusions. The city of Quixia, China, had ten times the incidence of stomach cancer as the community of Gangshan. The difference was found to be the custom in Gangshan to eat about seven cloves of garlic per day, while garlic was rarely eaten in Quixia. It is believed that garlic reduces the nitrites in the diet to prevent the formation of nitrosamines, which are powerful carcinogens. Dr. Sidney Belman is currently working on research in Japan to confirm this hypothesis. The Sloan Kettering Cancer Center in New York also has concluded that garlic inhibits the growth of cancer cells in the laboratory.

A List of Garlic's Myriad Benefits

Robert Crayhon summarizes garlic's many benefits:

1. Garlic has been shown to have powerful immune-boosting properties and may be valuable in fighting viral infections such as the common cold;

2. Garlic has been shown to help lower blood pressure in those with hypertension;

3. Garlic works as a natural antibiotic and reduces the number of harmful bacteria in the body;

4. Garlic reduces blood cholesterol and triglyceride levels and has been shown to limit the deposition of plaque on arterial walls;

5. Garlic has been shown to help the body eliminate parasites;

6. Garlic reduces the amount of yeast, *Candida albicans*, in the human GI tract and has been shown to be beneficial in fighting systemic yeast infections;

7. Garlic has been shown to lower blood sugar and to be of benefit to the diabetic;

8. Garlic has been shown in population and laboratory studies to help prevent a wide variety of cancers;

9. Garlic contains selenium, a cancer-preventing, immune-boosting, and anti-inflammatory nutrient.[25]

A Controversy Regarding Allicin

A controversy rages in the health industry regarding allicin. Allicin, found in raw garlic, is harsh, oxidative, and very unstable, and is a transient compound that rapidly decomposes to other compounds. It might be added that the credibility that garlic has enjoyed is in large degree due to the result of well over one hundred scientific studies that have been conducted on aged garlic extract and its constituents, not on allicin. The constituents that are unique to aged garlic extract include S-allymercaptocysteine and others. Those who insist that allicin is the key to garlic's potency will also insist that garlic should be eaten raw or lightly cooked. However, one researcher, Dr. Tariq Abdullah, reports that there was no difference between subjects who used raw garlic and those who used capsules in the power of their natural killer immune cells.

Garlic Appears to Work on Prostaglandins

What does appear to be important in garlic is that many of its components act on prostaglandins (hormonelike compounds), the fatty acids that regulate body functions like blood pressure, metabolism, and cell-division. When prostaglandins are overactive, they can cause hypertension, cancer, asthma, and excessive clotting. Garlic changes the way prostaglandins, are produced in the body so that they do not run out of control but maintain healthy functions.

Which Other Supplements Can We Use to Maximize Garlic's Effects?

There are other supplements that we can use synergistically to maximize garlic's effects. Omega-3 fatty acids (from fish oils) also suppress the production of prostaglandins and have similar effects on blood chemistry, immune system response, anti-inflammatory properties, and coronary disease reduction. Likewise, vitamin E inhibits prostaglandin, stimulates the immune system, and blocks the formation of nitrosamines. Vitamin C enhances the ability of vitamin E to do all of these things. Moderate exercise also strengthens immune response and has positive effects for the circulatory system.

Antioxidative Effects of Kyolic Garlic

S-allylcysteine—A Key Compound in Aged Garlic Extract (Kyolic Garlic)

"Though a plethora of compounds in aged garlic extract have demonstrated beneficial effects and a synergism of those compounds is likely responsible for the benefits of aged garlic extract for the sake of quality control, aged garlic extract is standardized with S-allylcysteine (SAC). SAC is a stable, effective, and safe organosulfar compound derived from garlic. A number of studies have shown that SAC can provide protection against oxidation, free radicals, pollution, cancer, and cardiovascular diseases. The bioavailability of SAC has been confirmed in several animals models."[26]

Lifestyle Shortcomings: Dr. Lau talks about the predicament that America faces. A similar one to other developed countries where countries become more wealthy, diseases of affluence such as heart attack, stroke, cancer, and diabetes increase. Those are all diseases that are the result of "lifestyle shortcomings." Further, he states that "[a] healthful lifestyle incorporating proper diet, exercise, rest, and effective stress management can contribute to rich, full life, as well as prevent a host of diseases." He continues that "[a]lthough many factors are involved in developing optimal health, some of which are beyond our control, such as 'hereditary factors,' there are many controllable factors including diet. One very simple food item which is receiving widespread recognition is the 'lowly garlic bulb.'" In his book, he shares with us the latest research findings on garlic and how it may retard or even reverse the aging process, restore memory loss, boost the immune function, nullify the effects of pollution, prevent cancer, reduce stress, and overcome allergy, among others.

Taken from *Garlic and You: The Modern Medicine*, by Benjamin Lau, M.D., Ph.D.

Garlic Inhibits the growth of Microbes and Bacteria: It was discovered that garlic is a potent broad-spectrum antibiotic. It inhibited the growth of a variety of microbes, including *Histoplasma capsulatum*, an important fungal pathogen in the central and eastern United States (also *Cryptococcus neoformans*, a yeast organism responsible for a very serious meningitis), and acid-fast bacteria, including species that cause tuberculosis.

His studies included the effect of garlic on *Candida albicans*, a yeast organism linked to the overuse of antibiotics. It was discovered that garlic acted on the lipid layer of the cell membrane, interfering with the lipid synthesis of this organism and other yeast organisms. In other words, the garlic caused these microbes to loose their membrane, the very lining of their bodies, which resulted in their inability to breathe. Interestingly, now it is known that garlic also inhibits animal cells, including human cells, from making lipids or fat molecules.

Taken from *Garlic and You: The Modem Medicine*, by Benjamin Lau, M.D., Ph.D.

Garlic and Viral Infections, AIDS: Viral infections also are positively affected by garlic. Dr. Lau describes how he knows many patients with chronic fatigue syndrome associated with the Epstein-Barr virus, the cytomegalo virus, the Coxsackie virus, and the herpes viruses that respond to garlic. Several studies have shown that garlic inhibits viral multiplication. In studies at the University of New Mexico Medical School, garlic was found to have antiviral activities against the influenza virus and the herpes simplex virus.

Dr. Lau states, "Garlic was also shown to potentiate antibody response in animals immunized with an influenza vaccine." A student working with Dr. Lau discovered that the human immunodeficiency virus (HIV), or AIDS virus, does not grow well in the presence of garlic in tissue culture. Further, he describes how "[a] colleague of mine, doing leprosy research, sent me a reprint showing garlic was successfully used in India for treating leprosy."

Taken from *Garlic and You: The Modem Medicine*, by Benjamin Lau, M.D., Ph.D.

Garlic and Amebic Dysentery: Another study at Tufts University revealed that garlic stopped the growth of *Entamoebia histolytica* that causes amebic dysentery. *Entamoebia histolytica* is a parasite that causes four million cases of dysentery diarrhea in the world each year. It is apparent that garlic has very potent antibacterial, as well as antiviral and antifungal, potential and is effective against viruses, bacteria, spirochetes, molds, yeasts, and parasites.

Taken from *Garlic and You: The Modern Medicine*, by Benjamin Lau, M.D., Ph.D.

Free Radicals and Major Diseases: "In this past decade, we have come to recognize that many acute and chronic human sufferings are the result of excess free radicals generated in our bodies."

Dr. Lau designates major illnesses associated with free radicals as "the four big As: arteriosclerosis, aging, allergies, and AIDS."

1. the four big As: Arteriosclerosis, Aging, Allergies, and AIDS;
2. blood pressure;
3. cancer;
4. inflammatory diseases such as arthritis, bronchitis, cystitis, and diverticulitis; and
5. chronic degenerative diseases such as MS, et cetera.

Taken from *Garlic and You: The Modern Medicine*, by Benjamin Lau, M.D., Ph.D.

Green Foods

Cereal Grasses

Cereal grass is the young green plant that grows to eventually produce the cereal grains (wheat, oats, rye, barley, and others). According to Ronald L. Seivolds's book *Cereal Grass: Nature's Greatest Health Gift* (Keats Publishing Inc., 1991), "[a]ll grasses look, smell, feel, taste, and most importantly have the nutrient and chemical make-up of green leafy vegetables, rather than of the cereal grains." He describes how the young cereal plant resembles long field grasses and that, for over fifty years, researchers have known that the cereal plant, at its young green stage, has many times the level of vitamins, minerals, enzymes, and proteins found in a mature cereal plant. The chemical and nutritional compositions of these young grasses differ greatly from those of mature cereal grain. The nutrients in the plant reach their peak values as they approach the brief and critical jointing stage. Seivolds describes this as, "[t]he stage representing the peak of the cereal plant's vegetative development." He claims that "the nutrient profile of cereal grasses is similar to those of the most nutritious dark green leafy vegetables."

A Powdered Extract Alternative

As a convenience food, a powdered extract of one of the cereal grasses, young barley grass, can be purchased in many natural health stores. This extract can simply be added to water to provide a quick dose of "liquid nutrition." Because dehydrated cereal grass compares favorably with other greens (with respect to both nutrients and cost), it is an excellent and convenient source of green food nutrients.

Green Foods Versus Processed Foods

If your mother told you to eat your vegetables, she was a wise woman. But when was the last time you did what your mother said? Unfortunately, today green foods have been pushed aside and processed foods have taken over.

The Protective Qualities of Natural Green Foods

It is well known now through modern research that green foods are rich in vitamins, minerals, and enzymes. They help protect against cancer, heart disease, digestive problems, and many other modern disorders. Green vegetables are excellent sources of complex carbohydrates, dietary fiber, beta-carotene, and chlorophyll. Possibly most important of all, they have potent antioxidant activity. Besides, they are low in fat and high in nutrients, an excellent combination.

Fiber-Rich Foods Protect Against Colon Cancer and Other Problems

It has been long known that fiber-rich foods protect against colon cancer, the second leading cause of cancer death in the U.S. Fiber is important in the digestive process in increasing the flow of saliva, decreasing the time that stools take to pass through the bowel, as well as increasing the frequency of elimination. Those of you who suffer from constipation, hemorrhoids, or colitis-type disorders would definitely benefit from a fiber-rich diet. Fiber is also very important as a "chelator," grabbing hold of toxins and eliminating them.

Man-Made, Processed Foods Generally Without Needed Fiber

One of the problems with processed foods is that the first thing they process *out* is the fiber. Canned vegetables are so overcooked that there are no vitamins and/or fiber left in them. Even "whole grain" breads contain processed wheat with a little of the bran put back. If we are to get the fiber we need from our diet, we have to eat whole foods.

Man-Made, Processed Foods Generally Without Phytochemicals

Phytochemicals are another important factor that processing elimi-nates. For years, nutrition researchers postulated that there were "associated food factors" that made whole, fresh foods better than processed foods. They insisted that vitamins were more effective when these other chemicals were not cooked out of the foods or processed out of the vitamins. They were scoffed at by the scientific community, who looked only at the chemicals in vitamins and told us that synthetic vitamins were just as good as natural ones. But in the last few years, these "associated food factors" have been iden-tified and researched, and their importance is now clearly recog-nized. Named phytochemicals as a group, they consist of thousands of chemicals such as flavonoids, carotenoids, tocopherols, and phe-nolic acids, each of which has antioxidant properties. Again, these important chemicals are found in the proper amounts and with the appropriate vitamins and minerals in whole, green foods. Live en-zymes are also among the chemicals "killed" by processing.

What Can Be Done?

Unfortunately, in our modern American society, for the majority of us whole green vegetables are not a large portion of our diets. There are a number of "green food supplements" that could fit into today's fast-paced lifestyle and can prove to be an excellent alternative to whole green vegetables.

Alfalfa Tablets

Alfalfa tablets were the first green food supplement to come on the market. Because of its deep root system (ten to twenty feet deep), many raw nutrients from mineral-rich soil are found in alfalfa. These include: vitamin A, pyridoxine (vitamin B_6), vita-min E, and vitamin K.

Green Barley, Wheat Grass, Spirulina, Chlorella, Aloe Vera, Jojoba, and Yucca

Other green food supplements include "baby" barley grass, wheat grass, spirulina, chlorella, aloe vera, jojoba, and yucca. All are high in vitamins, minerals, enzymes, fiber, and chlorophyll. Chlorophyll is sometimes referred to as the blood of plants.

Chlorophyll: Chlorophyll is a delicate, easily denatured element, held together by small bridges of magnesium. When it is heated, oxidized, or placed in an acidic environment, these bridges of magnesium begin to "fall out" and what remains is green pigment with very little, if any, nutritive value. For this reason, the best sources of chlorophyll are raw greens and Green Magma.

It is important to note that if chlorophyll is allowed to oxidize slowly, it forms a deadly toxin or by-product called pheophorbide (a photosensitizing agent capable of producing a fatal reaction). In Japan, the government has imposed stiff regulations governing the allowable amounts of pheophorbide in products containing chlorophyll. Before taking chlorophyll supplements, find out how far the processing plant is from the growing fields, the type of processing used (cooked, freeze-dried, or anything else), time elapsed from harvest to processing, and if alcohol or other acidic elements are added.

"Baby" Barley Grass

Among the most highly researched green food is "baby" barley grass. It is truly an ancient green food plant. Barley seeds have been discovered in Asia Minor dating back to 3500 B.C.E. Ancient historical records indicate that it was the first commercial crop and was the standard of currency in ancient Babylon. What? Barley was so important that it was used like money? Interesting. Barley is the world's oldest grain. It is known to have nourished the lake-dwellers of Switzerland a thousand years before Christ. Until the advent of wheat and rye, barley was the primary grain for bread in Europe.

World-famous researcher Dr. Yoshihide Hagiwara believes that green barley is the "ideal fast food" because the juice of the young green barley leaves contains potassium, calcium, magnesium, organic iron, copper, phosphorus, manganese, zinc, chlorophyll, and the important enzyme superoxide dismutase (SOD), all essential for good health. Green barley can be obtained in a tablet or powdered form sold as "Green Magma."

Professor Takayuki Shibamoto, Ph.D., chairman of the environmental toxicology division, University of California–Davis, has been studying a new antioxidant compound found in young green barley leaves called "2-0-GIV" (2-0-Glycosylisovitexin). 2-0-GIV is a flavonoid that inhibits lipid peroxidation (the formation of hydrogen peroxide in fat cells and tissues). According to Dr. Shibamoto, 2-0-GIV is as potent as any other antioxidant, including beta-carotene, vitamin C, or vitamin E. In one study reported in the *Journal of Agriculture and Food Chemistry* (1992), 2-0-GIV outperformed tocopherol (vitamin E). According to recent studies, green barley extract, in addition to its antioxidant activity, inhibits and reduces inflammation. Green barley helps those conditions which involve pain, swelling, heat, and redness. Therefore, it seems green barley would have application in a wide variety of inflammatory conditions.

The enzymes in green barley inactivate and break down carcinogens (*i.e.*, tobacco tar) as reported at the 102nd Annual Meeting of the Pharmaceutical Society of Japan. So, it acts as a cancer fighter as well.

Green barley extract has been shown to lower the rate of prostate cancer in the laboratory at George Washington Medical Center.

Green barley's circulatory benefits and its enhancement of the immune system have been known for some time and have been demonstrated in the clinical setting by Dr. Benjamin Lau, M.D., Ph.D., School of Medicine, Loma Linda University. His studies indicate that edible green plant extracts may serve as key preventive dietary supplements that enhance the immune system and prevent cancer (*International Nutritional Review*, July 1992).

Green Foods Help to Fight the Following Problems: Research also indicates that green foods may help fight the following:

- anemia
- arthritis
- asthma
- cancer
- constipation
- diabetes
- heart disease
- hypertension
- impotence
- obesity
- kidney disorders
- skin disorders

Green Magma

Green Magma, a green food made from "baby" barley grass, contains antioxidant vitamins C and E, as well as the newly discovered antioxidant compound 2-0-GIV. Additionally, Green Magma contains much chlorophyll; nineteen amino acids; beta-carotene; minerals; and the B vitamins, as well as very important live enzymes, including SOD (superoxide dismutase), a powerful antioxidant.

Green Magma is grown without pesticides or chemical fertilizers and is naturally processed. It is not a synthetic nutritional supplement, but a whole live food, a barley grass extract. I firmly believe whole live foods are a key to good health and long life.

Green Foods Company also produces "Wheat Germ Extract"; "Beta-Carrot" (a carrot juice powder); and "Green Essence," a "salad in a glass" that contains barley grass and other foods such as alfalfa, aloe, broccoli, celery, coix (perot barley), garlic, kelp, and spinach.

The Importance of Green Foods

The importance of green foods in the diet is now being validated scientifically worldwide. It is amazing how long it takes us to discover that foods were made correctly in the first place. They contain exactly what we need in their natural state. We have to find a way to take advantage of the whole foods naturally made, and most of us are not doing that presently with our diets. In fact, it would be difficult for anyone to eat enough green plants to equal the amount of nutrition in concentrated green food supplements. So, until you are ready to sidle up to a five-pound salad of spinach, watercress, alfalfa, and kelp, the concentrated supplements mentioned here are probably your best source for the vital nutrients you need from green foods.

Top Sources of Dietary Fiber:[27]
   Grains—all whole grains, including whole wheat, oatmeal, brown rice.
   Vegetables—acorn squash, beans (kidney, navy, pinto), broccoli, Brussels sprouts, cabbage, green peas, kale, radishes, spinach, winter squash, yams.
   Fruit—apples, blackberries, blueberries, pears, raspberries.
   The fiber present in whole foods is a mixture of soluble and insoluble fiber. A predominance of insoluble fiber is found in wheat bran. A pre-

dominance of soluble fiber is found in psyllium seed, apple pectin, and guar gum.

Beans supply about eight grams of fiber in a half cup (cooked). Most vegetables supply two to three grams of fiber in a half cup (cooked).

Top Dietary Sources of Antioxidants:[28]

Foods generally rich in antioxidants—red, yellow, and green vegetables, uncooked nuts and seeds (*e.g.*, almonds, Brazil nuts, hazelnuts, sunflower seeds), legumes, whole grains (*e.g.*, oatmeal and brown rice), garlic, shrimp, scallops.

Foods rich in carotenoids—apricots, broccoli, cantaloupe, carrots, collards, dandelion greens, kale, mustard greens, papaya, pumpkin, red peppers, sea vegetables (dulse, hijiki, kelp, nori, wakame), spinach, sweet potatoes, Swiss chard, tomatoes, winter squash.

Foods rich in bioflavonoids—beets, black cherries, blackberries, blueberries, cranberries, green asparagus tips, green tea, purple corn, purple onions, radishes, raspberries, red cabbage, red grapes, rhubarb, sweet potatoes, spices (ginger, parsley, rosemary, sage, thyme, turmeric).

Green Tea

What Is Green Tea?

Green tea is the antivirus, anticancer super antioxidant. It is the most popular of Asian drinks and has been known for centuries to have a long list of health benefits. Interestingly, after water, it is the most widely consumed beverage on the earth.

Dr. Earl Mindell states, "[t]he antioxidants specific to green tea are polyphenols, bioflavonoids that act as super antioxidants by neutralizing harmful fats and oils, lowering cholesterol and blood pressure, blocking cancer-triggering mechanisms, inhibiting bacteria and viruses, improving digestion, and protecting against ulcers and strokes. The specific type of polyphenol found in green tea is called a catechin."[29]

This catechin is similar to the substance found in grape seed extract that is the primary component of the proanthocyanadin molecule. The active polyphenols in green tea are the EGCG (epigallocatechin gallate).

Other ingredients in green tea include the green chlorophyll molecules, but also important are the proanthocyanadins similar to those found in grape seed extract, pine bark, bilberry, and gingko. The specific tea is a variety called *Camellia sinensis*.

Camellia sinensis in the West is known as black tea, such as Earl Grey tea, orange pekoe tea, or English breakfast tea.

What Are Some of Green Tea's Benefits?

Green tea inhibits cancer. Green tea protects the brain and liver. In one study, it was found to be two hundred times more protective against oxidation in the brain than vitamin E. Green tea is antibacterial. Green tea cures gum disease.

Green Tea Extract

Since green tea contains a significant amount of caffeine, and since ten to twenty cups a day would be necessary to take complete advantage of green tea's protective properties, a green tea extract in capsular form would be the preferred method of use. Dr. Mindell recommends two capsules of 30 percent polyphenol green tea extract daily with meals to control specific disease(s).

How Green Tea Can Help You

Dr. Earl Mindell in his *Super Antioxidant Miracle* book describes ways in which green tea could help you. These ways include protective safeguards against possible breast cancer, lung cancer, colon cancer, liver cancer, intestinal cancer, skin cancer, and stomach cancer. "Further," he states, "it prevents oxidation reactions in the brain, acts as an antibacterial against harmful digestive bacteria, it cures gum disease, it lowers oxidized LDL cholesterol and raises HDL cholesterol, it lowers triglycerides, inhibits viruses such as HIV, hepatitis, and herpes viruses, and acts as an antioxidant protectant against damage to blood vessels."[30]

The History of Green Tea

Legend has it that tea was first consumed as a beverage in 2737 B.C.E. when Emperor Shen Nung of the Tang Dynasty was watching a pot of boiling water and leaves from a nearby tree fell into the water. The aroma was so pleasant and enticing that he tasted it and never drank plain water again. About 800 C.E., Japanese priests studying in China learned of the drink and its medicinal properties from Buddhist monks and brought the practice back to their homeland. In the early 1200s, a book was written in Japan about tea drinking as a way to maintain health. It was not until 1609 that tea came to the West and found popularity in France, Holland, and Germany.

Where Does Tea Come From?

All tea comes from a single plant whose scientific name is *Camellia sinensis*, but this species has hundreds of variations dependent on geography, altitude, and soil conditions. The leaves may be picked at different stages, and there are also different ways of preparing the leaves. For our purposes, the difference between green teas and black teas is that black tea is allowed to ferment and is then fired to dry it out, whereas green tea is pan-fired *before* it has a chance to ferment. The fermentation process oxidizes some of the important bioflavonoids that give green tea its legendary ability to promote health and turns the leaves brown. The fresh, unoxidized green tea is the tea highest in antioxidants for this reason.

The Secret of Green Tea

The secret of green tea is the combination of flavonoids and polyphenols that it contains. There are three catechins that are especially noted for their effects. They are typically referred to as EC (epicatechin), EGC (epigallocatechin), and ECGC (epigallocatechin-3-gallate). Do not be overly concerned with all of these scientific terms. I include this type of detailed information for those of you wanting more in-depth knowledge. For most of us, the most important information to take from this section is that green tea contains numerous bioflavonoids (flavonoids, polyphenols, catechins), vitamins, and minerals that all work together synergistically when green tea is introduced into our bodies. In these subsequent paragraphs, I will be referring to green tea as a whole package, not just the individual parts.

Myriad Benefits Are Claimed

All kinds of benefits are claimed for tea, not the least of which is the simple fact that drinking a lot of tea keeps your urinary tract working. It also contains just enough caffeine to keep you stimulated (but not too high), lowers blood pressure by counteracting certain enzymes, lowers blood sugar, fights viruses and food poisoning, soothes digestion, and prevents cavities. That last one may be hard to swallow, but it was verified in December 1997 by some Japanese doctors who found out that if you just swirl green tea in your mouth, the chemicals stay in your saliva for up to an hour. Besides all that, it just feels good to hold a warm mug in your hands.

The Antioxidant Properties of Green Tea

The antioxidant properties of green tea are responsible for its most important benefits. The Chinese always claimed that tea slows aging, but it was not until we understood the role of oxidation in aging and the antioxidant function of flavonoids that we knew how this mechanism might work. In trying out a new computerized system for measuring chemicals, researchers at University of California–Berkeley found that green tea extract was *the best* at scavenging the deadly hydroxyl radicals. It was followed by grape seed extract, Pycnogenol, ginkgo biloba, and other commercial flavonoid blends. The three diseases that we will focus on regarding green tea are heart disease, AIDS, and cancer.

Heart Disease and the Benefits of Green Tea

Green tea, as we mentioned, lowers blood pressure. In the experiment that confirmed this, two groups of rats were used, and no matter which group got the tea extract, their blood pressure went down. In addition, the antioxidant effect of green tea stopped the oxidation of the "bad" LDL cholesterol and reduced lesions (wound or injury) in the aorta where oxidized cholesterol had started to plant itself. Neither vitamin E nor beta-carotene were as successful in that task. A few studies did not agree with this statement, but in the studies that confirm its antioxidant and cholesterol-lowering potential, there are key phrases like "there were no differences until week 11 . . ." and "women who drank 10 cups a day . . ." It is possible that results were not found because dosage was too low or not enough time was given. In one recent paper, the results are not in question:

Chinese green tea and Jasmine tea, both with a minimum degree of fermentation, were found to have significant serum and liver cholesterol lowering effects. They also reduced the increase in liver weight due to lipid deposition. All tea treatments lowered the atherogenic index and increased the HDL-total cholesterol ratio, while LDL-cholesterol and triglyceride levels were not significantly affected.[31]

That pretty much covers it all. The good cholesterol increased and the bad cholesterol did not do any bad things.

AIDS (Acquired Immunodeficiency Syndrome) and the Benefits of Green Tea

The idea that green tea could be used in treating AIDS is still in its infancy, but there are several indications that make it worth pursuing. First, green tea is known to inhibit viruses. Tobacco farmers use it to protect their crops from the tobacco mosaic virus. It is also known to directly attack the influenza virus. In 1990, green tea catechins were found to inhibit the activity of the AIDS virus in a laboratory petri dish. More recently, *Medical Hypotheses* published an article in March 1997 suggesting that several natural nutritional factors can prolong the effects of the new AIDS drug treatments. Those factors were selenium, a low-fat diet, green tea, and phytochemicals from cruciferous vegetables like turnips, cabbage, radishes, and horseradish. Also, if one of the key factors in controlling the progress of AIDS is controlling overall oxidative stress, then adding the antioxidant activity of green tea consumption should relieve much of that burden, keeping the disease in check.

Cancer and the Benefits of Green Tea

Most of the current research into green tea has focused on its cancer-fighting ability. As with other antioxidants, there is evidence to show that it stops the mutations in DNA that start cancer by scavenging the carcinogenic hydroxyl radicals and preventing damaging lesions where cancer likes to start. Tea catechins both reduce enzyme activity that can create free radicals and directly scavenge those particles. Like Pycnogenol, green tea also deals with the dangerous free radical nitric oxide and the enzymes that create it. There has been a surprising turn of events discovered in the last few months. In addition to these methods for combating cancer, green tea offers a new weapon: it tells mutant (cancer) cells to die!

Three studies published from November 1997 to March 1998 have independently cited evidence that green tea disrupts DNA replication and prevents the cancer cell from reproducing. The first was at Case Western Reserve University in Ohio, the second at Mie University in Japan, and the third at M. D. Anderson Cancer Research Center in Houston. The Case Western study saw something very unusual. The green tea catechins patched up the oxidative damage to the cell wall to keep the cancer cell from leaking and contaminating the cells around it, but some of the oxidative damage inside the cell was left untouched so that the cell would die quicker. Once that cancer cell died, it could be replaced by a healthy cell. This is a different approach, but one that is very effective. By forcing cancer cells to die early and stopping them from reproducing, the cancer cannot spread or grow and new tissue can grow in its place. The scientists call this stimulating cell "apoptosis" (programmed cell death).

Green tea has been associated with preventing several different kinds of cancer, including lung, breast, and stomach. That has now expanded to all of the digestive system cancers like those of the esophagus and colon. Since digestive cancers are responsible for one third of all the cancer deaths in the United States, green tea as a preventive measure could make a difference to thousands of people.

Lately, there have been several studies showing that tea catechins also help to prevent pancreatic cancer. In one case, the number of pancreatic cancers was cut in half in the group that received tea extract. Another study related this to specific antioxidant protection offered by tea catechins.

Green tea has also been shown to be effective in preventing cancer-causing UV (ultraviolet) radiation from mutating the DNA of skin cells. This is a concern because sunscreens do a great job of preventing sunburn, but do very little to block the frequencies of radiation that cause cancer, according to the Lovelace Institutes in Albuquerque, New Mexico.

Liver cancer was also affected by green tea in a study at Temple University. One of the more promising findings said that "EGCG [remember that stuff?] inhibited proliferation of AML [acute my-eloblastic leukemia] cells in *all* cases examined" [emphasis added]. It is almost impossible to find anything in medical research that works in all cases, so green tea holds great promise as a treatment for leukemia.

You may have noticed the phrase "tea catechins" used over and over again. What about all of the other components found in the tea? Some scientists in Osaka wondered the same thing, so they found out that the other chemicals are responsible for sup-pressing gene expression, inhibited the enzyme ornithine decar-boxylase, and stopped skin cancers from starting. Don't worry about the specifics in what all of those terms mean. Simply know and understand that all of that other "stuff" in green tea fights cancer in various ways as well. In fact, they found that these other polyphenols work in both the initiation phase and the promotion phase of cancer development, although there were several studies that indicated that the catechins were only effective in the promo-tion phase. Please translate this into English? Gladly. Research studies appear to indicate that *whole* green tea is more effective as a preventative measure to disease(s) than some of green tea's individual components (for example, catechins) if working alone. Suggestion? Drink green tea (or supplement with green tea ex-tract) and take advantage of *all* of its benefits.

Making the Decision to Drink Green Tea and/or Supplement Your Diet

If you really want to start supplementing with green tea, you should be aware that most of the successful experiments have a dosage equivalent to ten cups of tea a day. That is not impossible to do, but it takes a serious commitment to do it and a lot of trips to the bathroom. Pure extracts of green tea are readily available, which can significantly cut down the amount you have to drink. Also, this is a long-term lifestyle decision. The results are not seen over-night, even by the researchers who are looking for specific chemi-cal changes. It may take three months before you really see the benefits in terms of changes in disease status. What you will find right away is that you are getting about half as much caffeine as you get from coffee, your digestion will improve, and you will feel refreshed.

Herbs

Introduction

There are many herbs that contain antioxidants. The most potent of these herbal antioxidants are known as flavonoids, substances found in almost all plants. There are some who would go so far as to say that the flavonoids are even more potent antioxidants than vitamin E, and definitely more potent than vitamin C. According to Donald J. Brown in an article from *Herbs for Health*, Sept.–Oct. 1997, "four herbal antioxidants have been so extensively researched that we have established a general 'tissue-specific effect for them.' "[32]

Herbal Antioxidants and the Tissues They Protect		
Herbal Medicine	**Flavonoid (Antioxidant) Name**	**Tissues Protected**
Hawthorn	oligomeric procyanadins, vitexin	heart, circulatory system
Bilberry	anthocyanosides	eyes, circulatory system
Ginkgo	glycosides, ginkgolides, bilobasides	brain, nervous system, cardiovascular system
Milk thistle	silymarin	liver, gallbladder

"Beneficial effects of the flavonoids found in three herbs—gingko, bilberry, and milk thistle—are well documented. Hawthorn is not as well known to the general public, but research into its heart-benefiting antioxidant is promising, and may soon bring this herb into the spotlight."[33]

We will discuss in detail these four wonderful herbal antioxidants.

Hawthorn

Congestive Heart Failure and the Benefits of Hawthorn

I have had personal experience using hawthorn in a number of patients who suffered with cardiovascular disease, particularly congestive heart failure. In all instances, the congestive heart failure improved dramatically. One patient, a dear friend, suffered with cardiomyopathy with a functioning heart of less than 40 percent. Using a combination of hawthorn, vitamin E, and Co-Q-10, his cardiac function doubled, improving dramatically.

What Is the Hawthorn Plant?

The hawthorn plant thrives in the woodlands. It is a small shrublike tree with sharp thorns, and more than one hundred species of Crataegus are found throughout Europe, Western Asia, and North Africa.

Historically How Hawthorn Has Been Utilized

For centuries, hawthorn has been used to treat heart ailments, particularly "dropsy" (congestive heart failure). In addition, both Asian and European practitioners have used it for centuries to treat high blood pressure and angina pectoris. European researchers have discovered that the active ingredient in hawthorn is the oligomeric procyanidins, a complex of flavonoids. This flavonoid complex helps the heart pump more efficiently by increasing blood supply to the heart muscle through vasodilatation through the coronary arteries, increasing the heart's output of blood, and decreasing the peripheral vessel resistance, which improves blood flow. The overall result is a stronger, healthier heart with improved circulation.

For centuries, hawthorn extract has been known to be very effective in treating the early stages of congestive heart failure.

Hawthorn and Its Positive Effects on the Cardiovascular System

Hawthorn has proven to have very positive effects on the cardiovascular system. Dr. Daniel B. Mowrey suggests the following reasons: 1) peripheral vasodilatation, 2) dilation of the coronary arteries, 3) increased enzyme metabolism in the heart muscle, leading to better coronary health, and 4) increased oxygen utilization to the heart.

Hawthorn Berry Versus Digitalis: It is important for us to understand the difference between hawthorn berry and digitalis, the commonly used synthetic derivative of the *Digitalis perforia* plant, in the treatment of cardiovascular disease. Many of the undesirable properties of digitalis are antagonized by hawthorn. Further, hawthorn enhances pulse and positively potentiates the force of muscular contractions. Hawthorn differs from digitalis in that it lowers the blood pressure through vasodilatation, not through direct action on the heart. Hawthorn acts even on the healthy heart to increase cardiovascular activity. However, in heart disease, especially in cardiac insufficiency, according to Dr. Mowrey, "[h]awthorn appears to have a less immediate effect than digitalis.... Unlike digitalis, hawthorn exhibits an absence of cumulative activity. It appears to assume a position somewhere between digitalis and the potent adrenaline.... Another important finding is the apparent synergism between hawthorn berry and digitalis so that only about half of the dose of digitalis is required to obtain normal results."[34]

Bilberry

What Is Bilberry and Where Is it Found?

You may not have heard of the bilberry before. It is a cousin to the blueberry and the cranberry. In England it is called a whortleberry, the Scots know it as a blaeberry, and in America it is commonly called a huckleberry. But herbalists everywhere have agreed to call it a bilberry. It grows in many parts of Europe, but in North America it is limited to the mountains of British Columbia, Alberta, and south along the Rockies to Colorado.

World War II Royal Air Force Pilots Used Bilberry Jam for Night Vision

In World War II, the pilots of the Royal Air Force would eat bilberry jam on their bread before flying a night mission because they believed that it would improve their night vision. When the war was over, that prompted research that confirmed in 1964 that they were right.

What Is In Bilberry?

The "active ingredients" in bilberry are *anthocyanocides*. As you might guess, these are flavonoids closely related to the anthocyanidins of grape seed and pine bark extract. In fact, bilberry leaves are made up of more than 10 percent polyphenols (the flavonoid family that includes anthocyanocides). That is a lot of flavonoids! You know how bad blueberries can stain things, but they do not even compare with the amount of pigment (remember, flavonoids are pigments) in bilberries. The bilberry contains more anthocyanidins than any other fruit. The bilberry also contains the important antioxidant minerals zinc, manganese (used to build SOD), and selenium.

What Does Bilberry Do?

The main effect of bilberry is in improving circulation and blood vessel health, but the number one beneficiary of that action is your eyes. By preventing oxidative damage to the capillaries, it strengthens them to be more efficient, more flexible, and carry more oxygen to tissues. And bilberry does not stop with your capillaries; it strengthens arteries too, causing them to pump a little faster and a little harder. Bilberry also lowers blood pressure, reduces clotting, and contains glucoquinine, which can lower blood sugar.

How Does the Bilberry Help Your Eyes?

Your eyes are surrounded by tiny blood vessels that feed not only the tissues of the eyeball, but the nerves and muscles around your eye as well. More blood flow translates into more oxygen and nutrients coming into the eye and better removal of any wastes from that area. This means less stress to your eyes. In addition to that, bilberry helps to remove the oxidative stress that can damage both the vessels and the tissues of the eye. It just happens that the anthocyanocides in bilberry and the carotene lutein are the only antioxidants actually found inside the retina. These two actions (increased microcirculation and free radical scavenging) resolve the conflicts that cause most eye diseases.

Specific Eye Problems and the Benefits of Bilberry

Let's look at some of the causes of specific eye problems and how bilberry can help.

- *Cataracts*—This clouding of the lens is caused by oxidation and waste materials building up within it. Increased blood flow and free radical scavenging can stop this from happening. Reversal of cataract formation is possible in the early stages by using antioxidants (*i.e.*, bilberry).

* *Myopia* (nearsightedness)—Most myopia is caused by excessive stress in the muscles around the eye, usually occurring when reading in the dark, or just reading too much in grade school. So, you spend the rest of your life wearing glasses or contacts because of a temporary adjustment that your eyes made way back then. But bilberry can relieve the muscular stress enough to correct myopia or at least improve it significantly.

* *Pigmentary Retinitis*—One of the major symptoms of this disease is a limited field of vision or tunnel vision. Bilberry has helped these patients enlarge their field of vision and have better night vision.

* *Diabetic Retinopathy and Blindness*—There is nothing in this pathological "high sugar" condition that cannot be solved with bilberry. Diabetes causes microcirculation problems all over the body, both from constricted blood vessels and free radical damage. Even the issue of blood sugar control is aided by bilberry. In fact, bilberry has been shown to be the best hope available to diabetics facing vision impairment.

* *Glaucoma*—This is really a group of diseases that all result in degeneration of the optic nerve. Screening for this disease involves checking for changes in pressure inside the eyeball (that little puff of air the optometrist uses). Increased blood circulation and lowered blood pressure surely would relieve much of this problem, and antioxidant activity within the nerves of the eye could be expected to stop degeneration. The anthocyanadin family has the ability to pass through the barriers and get inside nerves as well as the brain.

* *Macular Degeneration*—This is one of the leading causes of blindness and is associated with both aging and smoking. The macula is that part of the retina where the light is focused after passing through the lens. When it degenerates, there is no stimuli sent to the rest of the nerves in the eye, hence no vision. Bilberry has proven effective in treating this disease because its principal cause is oxidative dam-

age. Bilberry also helps to deal with blue light, which is the frequency that causes the most damage to the eye.

Circulatory Problems and the Benefits of Bilberry

With all that it does for circulation, bilberry is now being used to treat circulatory problems, both in Europe and in the United States. Bilberry has also been shown to be helpful in treating ulcers since it increases the production of gastric mucous, which helps line the stomach.

Other Benefits of Bilberry

It is also helpful in healing wounds because it helps circulation to the wound, reduces oxidation, fights infection, and has the ability to cross-link with collagen to rebuild tissues. Recent research has also found it to inhibit certain enzymes that stimulate cancer growth.

Ginkgo

Where Does Ginkgo Come from and What Does it Do?

The ginkgo tree is the oldest species of tree still living on the earth. It is also one of the very few plants that is "sexual," the male flowers are found on one plant and the female fruits are on a different plant. One more thing: it stinks. Smells kind of like rancid butter. It has been used in Asia for over a thousand years to treat asthma, to aid digestion, and to prevent drunkenness. In China, they eat the cooked nuts (which are actually toxic, but apparently cooking kills the toxin) and describe how ginkgo helps bed-wetting and nocturnal emissions, eases bladder irritation, and brings back sexual energy. Most recently, studies have caused a great controversy about ginkgo as a brain stimulant, and possibly as a treatment for Alzheimer's disease.

Can We Inhibit the Aging Process on the Brain?

We can inhibit the aging process. The brain ages just as other organs do, but it does appear that the aging brain may be able to regenerate itself somewhat. Most important in keeping the brain young is that one must continue to challenge the function of one's brain. You need to continue to stimulate your brain through constructive mental activity. Resist being a "mental couch potato." Read books. Learn a foreign language. Take some classes. Do crossword puzzles. Just keep your brain working. Cleansing toxins from your system and moderate exercise will go a long way to help the brain improve its function, too. Possibly the most significant thing that any of us can do is to supply our brains with the supplements needed for peak function.

Is phosphatidylserine (PS) better than ginkgo for the anti-aging of the brain? Dr. Parris Kidd, an expert on aging, maintains that PS is the most universally beneficial of the anti-aging supplements. PS benefits memory, learning, concentration, word skills, mood, and coping with stress. Kidd says it is the only substance "proven to reverse brain aging" and that studies showing similar effects for ginkgo were flawed, not making distinction between improved circulation and brain function. PS is orthomolecular—that is, it normally occurs in the brain and is present in all brain cells—but ginkgo does not get into these cells. Because of this, PS is able to regenerate cell membranes and nerve cells that ginkgo cannot reach.

Kidd is probably right that ginkgo cannot have the profound regenerative effect that PS can have, being orthomolecular. However, his statements were made before the October 1997 study that was published in *JAMA* in which ginkgo was shown to improve cognitive performance in some patients and delay the progress of the disease by six months! And these were not patients with diagnosed cardiovascular disease. Ginkgo also has antioxidant activity that PS does not, due to its flavonoid constituents. It also does benefit circulation and blood flow because of the terpenes in it. For these reasons, it would seem best to use both PS and ginkgo for their different effects to treat impaired mental activity.

Ginkgo Biloba Extract

Ginkgo biloba extract is more an herbal preparation than a food. It is extracted from the leaves of the ginkgo tree. The word "biloba" means that these leaves have two lobes, like a couple of Japanese fans held together at the base. It has been used in Europe to help manage problems with circulation.

It is particularly helpful in increasing blood flow in the smallest blood vessels, the capillaries. It is here that toxins are likely to back up if there is not enough blood flowing through, but opening these pathways washes everything through and helps the body get rid of its poisons. If toxins are allowed to build up, free radicals build up, too, and damage the tiny capillaries and tissues they feed so that those organs cannot effectively do their job. For instance, your lungs take in air and hold it in minuscule sacs called alveoli, which feed the oxygen into the bloodstream through capillaries. If those capillaries are damaged by free radicals, or if the alveoli are damaged, it becomes extremely difficult to breathe. Ever heard of an asthma attack? The same is true for the fine network of tissues, nerves, and blood vessels in the eye. If toxins and free radicals back up, they can cause big problems, even blindness. Ginkgo can also benefit the small blood vessels that serve the ears and is one of the few promising treatments for tinnitus (ringing in the ears). It has also been shown to help restore circulation to areas of the brain damaged by stroke.

Ginkgo Has a Positive Effect in Dementia Cases

The big news for ginkgo came in October 1997 when the *Journal of the American Medical Association* published the results of a study that confirmed that ginkgo had a positive effect in cases of dementia. They used only patients whose main problem was mental impairment, whether someone had termed it Alzheimer's or not. They used every control imaginable and rated progress on three different scales to make sure that their results were accurate. Researchers even went so far as to switch everyone from the placebo to the real medicine and vice versa in the middle of the study. There is no doubt about it. Ginkgo stopped the progress of the disease in most cases, and many cases showed improvement. The effects were measurable at twelve weeks and noticeable at twenty-six weeks. Unfor-

tunately, almost half the people who started the study gave up before they reached that twenty-six-week mark. (Moral: Stick with it
and don't expect overnight results.)

Testing Cognitive Skills

Testing cognitive skills, the ginkgo group average showed very
little change from where they started, while the placebo group
grew decidedly worse in the same year. The scientists observed
that ginkgo delayed the progress of the disease by six months to a
year.

On another scale, measuring more social and functional skills,
the ginkgo group improved by almost the same amount that the
placebo group had deteriorated! The two lines on the chart were
like a reverse image of each other, one going up and the other
sliding down. For anyone who has had to help a parent dress
himself or herself or go to the bathroom simply because the elderly appear to forget what they are doing in the process, those
kind of results hold tremendous hope. Even though scientific researchers reported that the disease was delayed by six months to
a year, the study lasted only a year. The long-term findings are not
in yet.

The Degree of Severity of Mental Impairment Did Not Matter

Researchers also found that it did not matter how severe the problem was when the patient started treatment. Whether the patient
already had severe impairment or had just noticed that he was
experiencing some trouble finding the word he was searching for,
the progress of the disease stopped, and about the same amount
of improvement was seen in everyone. That did not make the
most severe cases just like the less severe ones, but their overall
improvement *from where they had been* was about the same.

German Studies Had Already Proven that Ginkgo Works

This research was designed to find out if ginkgo really worked.
Actually, the American researchers admitted in their introduction
that German studies had already shown that it worked, but Americans are stubborn and do not believe anything until they try it

themselves. What they did not try to find was *why* it worked or *how* it worked. American researchers did offer this suggestion:

> ... [t]he main effects seem to be related to its [ginkgo's] antioxidant properties, which require the synergistic action of the flavonoids, the terpenoids (ginkgogolides, bioalide), and the organic acids, principal constituents of [ginkgo extract]. These compounds to varying degrees act as scavengers for free radicals, which have been considered the mediators of the excessive lipid peroxidation and cell damage observed in Alzheimer's disease.[35]

Start Preventive Measures Today!

You don't have to wait until you start forgetting your zip code. If the enemy is oxidative damage, stop it now, before it accumulates and causes more problems. What is the worst that could happen? The blood flow to your brain would increase and you would remember things better and think faster. Terrible! You might even be more alert and be in a better mood. Oh, it could be disastrous if that happened. You just might even keep your mental faculties sharp all the way into old age and enjoy life without the frustration of being confused all the time or the guilt of being a burden on loved ones.

Asthma, Allergies, and the Benefits of Ginkgo

I was not joking about asthma. Aside from preventing free radical damage, ginkgo relieves the effects of asthma and allergies by blocking a chemical called PAF (platelet activating factor). PAF is released as a normal immune system response when the situation calls for blood to clot, infection to localize a germ, or mucous membranes to secrete. But your body can overreact. When it does overreact to things like dust or pollen, we have an allergic response. We secrete too much mucus in our nose and throat, our bronchial tubes tighten up so we cannot breathe, and you would logically think you had a sinus infection when it is actually a little dust in your nose. In asthmatics, the same response leads to a crisis situation because breathing is already difficult and the reaction goes all the way into the lungs. Ginkgo blocks PAF so it can't overreact. By normalizing this reaction, allergic and asthmatic episodes are less frequent, less severe, and might be eliminated. It is probably best to take ginkgo long term for this condition since you never really know when you might encounter a problem situation.

Eye Damage and the Benefits of Ginkgo

The part about eye damage is real, too. A Swedish study showed that ginkgo improved the distance-vision of people who already showed signs of degeneration in the retina. The disease macular degeneration, a leading cause of blindness, is strongly related to hemorrhages in the fine blood vessels in the eye, possibly due to oxidative stress. By strengthening the tiny blood vessels in the eye, and by acting as an antioxidant, ginkgo provides a double whammy against eye diseases.

Ginkgo Tea or Ginkgo Biloba Extract

It is possible to prepare tea from ginkgo leaves, but remember what I said about the tree: it stinks. So maybe a standardized extract is a better solution. A dosage of 80 to 150 milligrams a day is normal. The dosage used in the dementia experiment was 40 milligrams three times a day (120 milligrams total).

Milk Thistle

Milk Thistle (Silymarin) Saved the Day!

I believe that silymarin saved the life of a dear friend of mine, an alcoholic for a number of years. When he finally stopped drinking, his liver had been so damaged that many of us were fearful he would die from liver failure in spite of controlling his terrible addiction.

Silymarin saved the day. Of course, there were other things that were done, but in my opinion, this marvelous herb reversed the damage that alcohol had done to his liver.

What Is Milk Thistle and What Does it Do?

Milk thistle acquired its name from the milky sap that comes from its leaves and stems. Although known for centuries as a liver medicine, only in the past two decades has the active ingredient, silymarin, a group of flavonoid compounds, been discovered. These compounds have a remarkable effect in protecting the liver from oxidant damage (as an antioxidant) and in enhancing the liver's detoxification processes. In 1968, a group of German researchers identified a flavonoid complex in the milk thistle seed that they ultimately christened silymarin.[36] Silymarin raises glutathione levels in liver cells by as much as 50 percent. Further, these German researchers state that silymarin also "[i]ncreases the activity of another antioxidant, superoxide dismutase, in blood cells."[37]

We discussed in the cancer section the importance of the liver in the detoxification process. In this section, we will concentrate more on its importance as an antioxidant.

Milk Thistle (Silymarin) Prevents Damage to the Liver

Silymarin prevents damage to the liver because it acts as an antioxidant.[38] Far more potent in antioxidant activity than either vitamin E or vitamin C, silymarin seems to be very specific in its antioxidant activity in the liver.

As is commonly the case in the plant kingdom, the flavonoids work along with vitamin C, producing many health benefits. In fact, the flavonoids have been considered as a vitamin, even being called vitamin P by some researchers.

One of the key ways in which silymarin enhances the liver detoxification reaction is by preventing the depletion of the important glutathione, which is linked to the liver's ability to detoxify. Simply put, the higher the glutathione level in the liver, the greater the liver's capacity to detoxify the body. Reduction of glutathione renders the liver cell vulnerable to damage.

A most interesting study presented in *Planta Medica* showed that silymarin not only prevents the depletion of glutathione, but has been shown to increase the level of glutathione of the liver by up to 35 percent.[39] Logically, we could then say that silymarin can increase liver detoxification by up to 35 percent. I certainly observed this in my alcoholic friend and his recovery.

The Liver Is Vitally Important in Detoxifying Poisons in Our Bodies

The liver is so very important in detoxifying poisons that enter our bodies, breaking down potentially lethal substances such as alcohol, nicotine, air and water pollutants, and varied carcinogens. Incredible! You certainly can understand why it is important to keep your liver in as good a working condition as humanly possible in today's pollution-riddled environment. Remember also that vitamins A, D, E, and K are all stored in the liver.

How Milk Thistle (Silymarin) Inhibits Liver Damage

In conclusion, here is what Dr. Michael Murray has to say about silymarin and how it inhibits liver damage by the following actions: "[silymarin] acts as a direct antioxidant and free radical scavenger. It increases the intracellular levels of glutathione and superoxide dismutase. It inhibits the formation of leukotrienes (inflammatory compounds when produced when oxygen interacts with fatty acids). It stimulates hepatocyte regeneration."

Additionally, Dr. Murray refers to a new form of silymarin that is bound to phosphatidylcholine, referred to as silymarin phytosone. "A growing body of scientific research indicates that silymarin phytosone is better absorbed and produces better clinical results than unbound silymarin."[40]

Recommended Dosages and Specifics About Milk Thistle (Silymarin)

Silymarin is nontoxic, but since it does increase bile flow, it may produce a mild laxative effect and a looser stool.

One should look for a standardized preparation of 70 to 80 percent silymarin. As a preventive measure against liver damage, it is suggested that you take three 160-milligram doses a day for six to eight weeks. After that, the dosage can be lowered to 280 milligrams a day.

Milk Thistle: To most people, milk thistle is an ugly, bristly, prickly weed that can quickly take over a field or a garden. But to anyone with liver problems, it can be a beneficial tool in fighting cirrhosis, hepatitis, jaundice, and the effects of alcohol and drug abuse.

The silymarin compounds in milk thistle are powerful antioxidants that protect the liver from cell damage caused by free radicals. As a preventative measure against liver damage, it is suggested that you take three 160-milligram doses a day for six to eight weeks. After that, the dosage can be lowered to 280 milligrams a day.

In addition to liver problems, milk thistle can be effective in treating lesser problems linked to digestion. Whenever you have digestive problems brought on by eating too much or by eating the wrong combination of foods, try taking a tablet of concentrated milk thistle powder three times a day for several days. When purchasing milk thistle at your local natural or health food store, look for standard preparations that are 80 percent silymarin.

Melatonin

The Pineal Gland

Almost perfectly in the center of your brain is a tiny gland that, as late as the 1960s, was considered to be inactive. It was seen as a benign remnant of some evolutionary process. It is called the pineal gland because it is shaped somewhat like a pine cone. Now we know that this little pine cone may be the most important gland in your body. The pineal controls the other glandular systems, and in doing so, controls the immune system, the reproductive system, sleep patterns, and most importantly, the aging process. This is all done through melatonin, a hormone that the pineal produces in almost undetectable amounts.

Your Biological Clock

You know that biological clock that people keep telling you is ticking? The pineal gland is it! Walter Pierpaoli, one of the foremost researchers of melatonin and co-author of *The Melatonin Miracle,* says,

> We discovered that the pineal gland is to our bodies what the conductor is to the orchestra. The job of the pineal gland is to regulate and harmonize the functioning of a number of bodily systems. One of those systems is our endocrine system, which is made up of many glands that produce hormones that control our growth from childhood to adulthood. They also control our

sexual development. Another of these systems is the immune
system, which protects us against disease. In its capacity as the
regulator of these systems, the pineal also functions as the body's
aging clock. When the pineal begins to run down, so do all the
other systems under its control.[41]

What Is Melatonin and Where Is it Found?

Melatonin is chemically related to both melanin, a skin pigment,
and serotonin, a neurotransmitter in the brain associated with
good, happy feelings. In addition to being produced by the pineal
gland, it is also produced constantly in the digestive tract. This
occurs independently of the pineal gland and establishes a baseline
amount of melatonin for your body to use. Melatonin can be
found virtually everywhere in your body, in every cell. For years,
medical researchers knew it was there, but did not know what it
did. It turns out that, ounce for ounce (or microgram for microgram in this case), melatonin is the most powerful antioxidant we
have found!

Before we talk about melatonin's effects as an antioxidant,
let's make sure you understand how it works as the master gland.
The pineal is activated by light and is directly connected to your
eyes. When you open your eyes in the morning and get that first
burst of sunlight, the pineal gland gets the signal to begin its day,
and the first activity is to shut down the production of melatonin.
Shortly after darkness falls, the pineal releases melatonin to prepare for sleep. The ancient Chinese even called the pineal the "third
eye" because of this sensitivity. This cycle and the way it adjusts
to seasonal changes is known as our circadian rhythm. Left to
itself, in subjects isolated from light for long periods of time, the
pineal establishes a cycle of about twenty-five hours for activity,
sleeping, and waking. This cycle can be adjusted about two to
three hours either way by light and dark input, so that seasonal
adjustments or trips across a couple of time zones do not affect us
much. But when we mess up the cycle with an erratic schedule or
a trip that crosses several time zones (especially west to east), it is
harder for the pineal to adjust, and we may find ourselves wide
awake when we want to sleep or sleepy all day long. That may
get the pineal gland really confused, which in turn creates havoc
in the other systems it controls. This may be why we are more

susceptible to diseases when we do not get enough sleep: In essence, our immune system has not received the right signals from the pineal gland. If that kind of crazy schedule is kept up for a long period of time, this can lead to some serious problems.

Melatonin in Mid-Life

One more thing: the pineal begins to cut back production of melatonin in mid-life, between the ages of forty and fifty. After a few years, it begins to calcify and eventually shuts down completely. In some people of advanced age, the pineal appears to be a little rock in the middle of their heads. This is a key event in the aging process. At that point, the immune system begins to falter, incidence of cancer increases, energy begins to decline rapidly, and sleep becomes increasingly irregular. It may even explain the graying of hair.

You are going to wonder what all this has to do with antioxidants for the next few pages. Trust me; we'll get to that eventually.

The Pineal Gland and Your Immune System

Let's back up and talk about how the pineal is connected to the immune system. The thymus is the gland that makes T-cells for the immune system. One of the peculiar things about the thymus is that it grows normally through puberty and then begins to shrink, sometimes disappearing completely. Unfortunately, when it disappears, so does its function as an immune booster, which is why older people have less resistance to certain diseases, especially cancers. The thymus is also connected to the pituitary, which produces growth hormone. When the thymus starts shrinking, growth tends to stop also. In mice where the thymus was removed shortly after birth, they grew very quickly, but also grew old and sick very quickly, having almost no immune system. However, the same type of mice would grow normally in a sterile "bubble" where they were not exposed to disease. That meant the thymus only related to the immune system and could not be the gland that controlled development and aging. So, what was the controller?

More experiments showed that the thymus was connected to the thyroid (which regulates both growth and immune responses), the hypothalamus (which regulates the pituitary), and the adrenal glands (which stimulate the sex hormones). It was clear that all of these glands controlling growth, immunity, and reproduction were communicating to each other, even though previous theories had said these systems were autonomous and independent. Eventually, Pierpaoli noticed that the results of one experiment were dependent on the time of day in which treatment was given.

Circadian Rhythms Might Hold the Answer

This began his studies into how circadian rhythms, already known to be controlled by the pineal gland, might hold the answer to his questions.

Upon learning that blind people (who have no sensitivity to light) lived longer than those who had some light sensitivity, he got the idea that light might affect longevity. He started raising mice in an environment of constant artificial light with no "night." The first three generations developed normally, had normal immune response, reproduced, and lived out their expected lifespan.

> By the fourth generation, however, the difference in the mice was striking. The mice no longer looked like healthy mice: Their muscles began to shrink, they grew wrinkled, they developed bald patches on their fur, their thymus glands (where T-cells are stored) developed fatty tissue, and their immune response was poor. They looked like tired little old mice. . . . When we kept mice under continuous light so that their melatonin production was decreased and erratic, their immune function was depressed and they aged prematurely and died young. In addition, within four generations they stopped reproducing altogether.[42]

Is the Amount of Melatonin Produced in the Pineal Gland the Key?

Suddenly there was a definite and clear connection between the immune system, the endocrine system, and the reproductive system, and it was rooted in the work of melatonin. To verify this theory, the pineal glands of young mice were cross-transplanted with the glands of older mice. The young mice with old pineal glands began to age rapidly and become sick. The old mice that had young pineal glands did just the opposite: They became stronger, healthier, and more youthful in appearance. Pierpaoli relates that one day he walked into the laboratory and realized that the two groups of mice looked as if they were the same age, even though they were born fourteen months apart (the equivalent of about forty human years). That is like a forty-year-old and an eighty-year-old looking the same age! The only possible explanation was that the younger, more productive pineal glands rejuvenated the old mice, while the pineals from those old mice caused the young mice to develop all the signs of aging. All of this related specifically to the amount of melatonin produced by the pineal glands.

Can We Reset our Biological Clocks?

Now the question is: Can we reset our biological clocks? Can we restore youthfulness, immune response, and sexual response? The answer appears to be yes, at least in a limited way. As our understanding grows, we may be able to change those limitations. As we age, the different systems tend to lose their ability to work together as the pineal degenerates. Melatonin supplementation appears to prevent this state of disorder by reconnecting these systems so that they can work in harmony with one another. With what we know so far, we can at least begin to control some of the effects of aging, such as declining immune function, sleep disorders, heart disease, and susceptibility to cancer.

Melatonin Supplements and Boosting the Immune System

To boost the immune system, melatonin supplements can actually grow back a withered thymus gland, restoring T-cell function. Melatonin supplements taken an hour or two before bedtime stimulate the natural release of the hormone and help you get to sleep and stay asleep until morning. It also has a normalizing effect on cholesterol and blood pressure, bringing down high levels in both measures of heart disease. By restoring the immune system, it enables the body to seek and destroy mutant cells before cancers can develop, and it reduces the effectiveness of certain hormones that cause breast and prostate cancers to spread.

Melatonin in the digestive tract also helps the body absorb zinc, which is essential to the immune system but hard for older people to get enough of. All those wonderful attributes, and we have not yet addressed its antioxidant capabilities.

Melatonin as an Antioxidant

As an antioxidant, melatonin is unique in several ways. As we mentioned, it is found in almost every cell in your body. It is fat-soluble, so it slips right through cell membranes, and its favorite place to be found is around the nucleus of the cell (where the DNA is stored). It is especially effective against the hydroxyl radical. Most importantly, after neutralizing free radicals, it remains stable and does not need to be restored, as most other antioxidants do.

Let's put all of that together: It is the most effective antioxidant against the worst type of free radical, it is in every cell, it stays in the cell walls and around the DNA where it is needed most, and it remains stable at all times. Sounds great to me.

Melatonin and the Energy Producer in Our Human Cells

Also, it has a special relationship with the mitochondria of the cell. Remember that the mitochondria are the energy producers of the cell and of the body. They produces a fuel called ATP, which your body burns as fuel. By regulating certain functions of the thyroid gland, melatonin regulates the release of the energy to the mitochondria and then from the mitochondria to different organs in the body. Along the way, it also works as an antioxidant to soak up the free radicals produced as the mitochondria metabolize oxygen to make ATP. So, it tells the mitochondria to start working, takes care of the problems caused by their work, and then distributes their product to the rest of the body. The bottom line is that you have more energy to do the things you want to do. The younger you are, with more melatonin, the more energy you have. If you are not so young and your pineal gland has started to slack off, more melatonin can restore your energy levels and make you feel younger.

Memory loss is one effect of aging that many people dread. The amino acid glutamate is normally a good guy that helps us establish pathways in the brain that organize our thoughts, actions, and memories. However, with time these pathways can get worn out. The constant electrical pulses that fire across the synapses of the brain can turn these pathways into ruts. Those thought patterns or habits that we follow the most are the ones most likely to become overworked. The electrical pulses themselves produce free radicals that can damage the nerves along that pathway. Then the glutamate that established the pathway also produces free radicals. The end result is that the things most familiar to you can become foreign because that overworked pathway has disintegrated and your thought literally gets lost, not knowing where to make the next connection. The more fixed we have been in our thinking, the more that we have done by habit or repeated over and over, the greater the danger of degeneration in these neural pathways.

Melatonin and the Brain

But if we replace the melatonin that the pineal used to produce, it will clean up the free radicals and keep our mind fresh and our nerve cells intact. It even encourages the establishment of alternate pathways so that the old pathways do not become overused. Maybe you *can* teach an old dog new tricks!

Melatonin and Cancer

Melatonin's effects in preventing and treating cancer may be its most significant contribution. Research going back to 1940 showed that something made by the pineal gland could stop cancers from growing and that removing the pineal made cancers grow faster. They just did not know what it was. Another mystery was why blind women were only half as likely to get breast cancer as sighted women. Is it the melatonin level? (Blind people never have daylight shut down their pineal gland.) We have now conducted tests that confirm that melatonin slows the growth of cancer cells *in vitro* and in mice. In one study, the growth of an aggressive skin cancer (melanoma) was slowed by a factor of five, and its spreading was delayed.

We mentioned before that melatonin fights cancer by stimulating the immune system to kill cancer cells before they replicate and by regulating hormones that might cause cancer to spread. The third way melatonin fights cancer is as an antioxidant, protecting cells from oxidative damage. The two places in the cell where melatonin is most likely to be found are the cell wall and the nucleus. These are exactly the places where free radicals are most likely to cause the kinds of damage that lead to cancerous growths. Melatonin stands as a watchdog over the cell's genetic code, ready to protect it from invaders.

Interleukin-2, Melatonin, and Cancer

One of the more promising treatments for cancer in the last decade has been interleukin-2 (IL-2), a substance made by the immune system that detects cancer cells and calls the immune system into action. The great drawback to its use has been the extremely harsh side effects, which made some of the early testers so violently ill that they died. Those side effects seem to be eased when a smaller dose of IL-2 is given along with melatonin. Dr. Steven Bock reports this study:

> A group of researchers at San Gerardo Hospital in Monza, Italy, conducted tests to see if melatonin could enhance the effectiveness of IL-2 against other cancers as well. They administered low doses of IL-2 (to reduce the severe side effects) with melatonin to 82 patients, most of whom had metastases, that is, cancer that had spread from its initial site to distant organs. The regimen shrank the tumors in 21 of the patients. Side effects were mild in all the patients. Another experiment by the same group found that melatonin significantly improved the effectiveness of IL-2, seven percent of patients receiving both melatonin and IL-2 experienced complete remissions, versus none in the group receiving IL-2 alone. Twenty percent of those receiving the combination therapy had partial remissions, versus three percent of those who received only IL-2. Survival after one year was 46 percent for the first group, versus only 15 percent for the IL-2 only group.[43]

Think about that. The survival rate was three times higher and the chances of complete remission went from none to some! That is significant. Best of all, the side effects did not make the patients miserable. With this kind of start, imagine what kind of results are possible when we learn more about this combination!

Melatonin and Electromagnetic Field Radiation

There has been some speculation that melatonin would also help reduce free radical damage from a type of radiation known as EMF (electromagnetic field) radiation. There has been some debate about whether this type of radiation even exists, but most of the objections have been raised by industries that depend on machinery that produces the problem. Any electrical motor produces an electromagnetic field, as do power lines, TV screens, computers and monitors, and the wiring in your house. One of the worst offenders is your electric blanket. It puts out a level of radiation that is about four times the acceptable level, and you stay wrapped up in it, no more than a couple of inches away from it, for six to eight hours every night.

EMF radiation from high-tension power lines and converters has been linked to an increase in leukemia and a variety of cancers in the people who live under them. These are not the lines that carry power through your neighborhood. Most of those are low-tension lines that only generate a low-level EMF reading. The big main lines that carry power between communities are the problem. As we learned more about melatonin, it became clear that the list of cancers caused by EMF radiation and the list caused by low melatonin levels looked a lot alike. Is it possible that EMF radiation was causing low melatonin levels?

It is really quite likely. We tend to think of radio waves, light, and magnetic fields as totally different kinds of energy, but they are really exactly the same kinds of waves at different frequencies. That is why microwave ovens work. The sound waves they generate heat objects in exactly the same way that light, radiant heat, or radiation from a nuclear explosion would. Since the pineal shuts down when waves in the range of visible light hit the eyes, it would not be too surprising that waves in other ranges might have the same effect, even if our eyes cannot detect them. Several studies have now confirmed that both animals and humans exposed to EMFs for about twenty hours a day will find that their pineal gland has almost shut down completely. When the radiation is removed, melatonin levels go right back to normal within a few days.

Probably those guys who said EMF radiation is too weak to do enough damage to cause cancer were right. But if EMF radiation shuts down our pineal gland, it shuts down our immune system as well. Weakened immune systems cause cancer. Once the immune system is weak, there is no way to fight off the damage that free radicals are causing with or without the help of radiation.

A Review of the Benefits of Melatonin

Let's review again for a moment. Melatonin regulates the immune system, the reproductive system, and the endocrine system, as well as controlling our sleep cycles. It is found everywhere in your body and acts as an antioxidant in the cells. By stimulating the thymus, it controls the part of the immune system that determines when and where to attack. As the pineal shuts down in mid-life, symptoms and diseases begin to appear that we associate with aging but that are really signs of a weakened immune system, the system the pineal gland formerly regulated. As we put all the puzzle pieces together, it is clear that the role played by the pineal gland is extremely important to the immune system. But some have gone a step further. There is some speculation that the pineal also controls the entire antioxidant system, which actually is a subsystem of the immune system anyway. Maybe this *master gland* is also a *master antioxidant*. Maybe that is why it is found all over your body and not just in the glands. No, we do not have adequate research to back up that hypothesis yet, but it is worth pursuing.

Now for the big question: Does this mean that we can stop the aging process by taking melatonin? Probably not. Most evidence says that life span is set by a number of different genetic factors. But that doesn't mean we have to be unduly sick as we age. What melatonin can do is reduce the risks of the diseases associated with aging and make our later years a lot more fun. Instead of watching ourselves shrivel up and waste away, we can stay healthy, retain muscle mass, be more active, and keep our minds sharper. Melatonin supplements have only been used in humans for a few years, so we have not had sufficient time to see exactly what effects it will have on people who begin taking it in their forties and keep it up into their eighties. But do you really want to wait another thirty-five years before you start taking it yourself?

Recommendations and General Cautions About Taking Melatonin

Melatonin seems to be a very safe supplement, but there are some cautions you should know about. First, more is not necessarily better. A low dose is fine; usually 1 to 3 milligrams taken a couple of hours before bedtime is all that is needed. If you are over sixty-five, you may want to go to as much as 5 milligrams, but start slowly and work up to it. Taking more does not make it work better, and since it is fat-soluble, it might build up in fat cells. Of course, you can do a lot to help out your pineal gland by keeping a regular schedule that mirrors the cycle of the sun, getting up somewhere around daybreak and going to bed a few hours after nightfall.

You should not take melatonin without consulting your doctor if:

1. You are taking any medication that affects the same systems that melatonin affects. If you are already taking medication to boost your immune system, boost serotonin levels, lower blood pressure, or increase hormones, there will probably be a conflict with melatonin. Even aspirin, birth control pills, Prozac, Valium, or thyroid medications can cause conflicts. Check with your doctor first.

2. You already have cancer, hormonal disorders, depression or other psychiatric disorders, allergies or autoimmune disorders, or fertility problems, or you are nursing a baby. All of these conditions indicate a problem in the systems regulated by the pineal and more melatonin could get your body really confused.

3. You are a child or adolescent. Really, you should not even be thinking about melatonin unless you are over forty. Young people have perfectly good pineal glands that produce plenty of melatonin for them. If you are under forty and really think you might need melatonin, you probably just need to adjust your schedule, activities, and diet to give your pineal gland some help. Get a book on the sub-

ject and follow its recommendations, but do not start taking pills that you do not really need.

Melatonin and Sex

One last word about melatonin: sex. Melatonin stimulates testosterone, estrogen, and adrenaline to extend your sex life and
make it better. If that doesn't sell you on it, you're dead already.

5-HTP

5-HTP Is Also a Potent Antioxidant

According to Dr. Michael Murray, 5-hydroxytryptophan (5-HTP)
is also a potent antioxidant.[44] Although its prime function is as a
building block of serotonin, the neurotransmitter that tends to
regulate moods, appetites, and sleep patterns, it, in addition, can
prevent damage to the body caused by free radicals, which includes reducing the risk of serious illnesses such as cancer.

I was intrigued as I read this work first because of my little
knowledge of serotonin, the important neurotransmitter that regulates as a chemical that carries essential signals from one brain
cell to the other, as Dr. Murray describes it, "a master control
chemical" of the brain. What I had not understood before was its
important connection to the overall immune system of the body:
that 5-HTP increases melatonin production, as well as raising the
levels of endorphins, the body's natural defense against stress and
mild pain.

Since 5-HTP, the precursor of serotonin synthesis, I discovered that certain supplements enhanced the production of 5-HTP
and supported this serotonin synthesis. First were the B vitamins
that were needed for serotonin synthesis. Additionally there are
vitamin C, vitamin E, and beta-carotene as the precursor for vitamin A. It is obvious that a good multivitamin is extremely important. In addition, since magnesium, manganese, potassium,
selenium, copper, zinc, chromium, and calcium are considered
important minerals in the overall synthesis of serotonin, it is obvious that all of these vitamins and minerals are extremely important in the overall synthesis of serotonin from 5-HTP.

Probably most important is Dr. Murray's recommendation that extra antioxidants be taken because low intake of antioxidants results in decreased serotonin levels. Conversely, keeping one's antioxidant intake high can help you maintain your serotonin level.[45]

A Combination of Antioxidants Proves to Be Greater Protection

Dr. Murray states, "[e]xtensive research shows that a combination of antioxidants provides greater protection than does taking a high dose of any single antioxidant. Mixtures of antioxidant nutrients appear to work together harmoniously to produce the phenomenon known as synergy, where the whole is greater than the sum of the parts. In other words, when it comes to the benefits of antioxidants, one plus one equals three."[46]

B Vitamins and 5-HTP: The first symptoms of a subclinical nutritional deficiency are often psychological. It has been my opinion that the B vitamins are the single most important vitamins for the brain. For instance, folic acid and B_{12} are two nutrients generally working together as a team. Your body must have proper amounts of both to convert 5-HTP into serotonin.

Vitamin B_6 is also very much involved in the manufacture of the neurotransmitters, including serotonin.

The B vitamins important here are: vitamin B_1 (thiamine), vitamin B_2 (riboflavin), vitamin B_3 (niacin), vitamin B_5 (pantothenic acid), vitamin B_6 (pyridoxine), and vitamin B_{12} (biotin and folic acid).

Minerals

Along with vitamins, our bodies also need trace amounts of minerals. Most of us have heard of some of the minerals we need from commercials about "iron-poor blood," cough drops with zinc, and "calcium for strong teeth and bones." (Oops, I think that was a dog biscuit commercial.) Other minerals that you need, but may not have heard about, are manganese, copper, iodine, magnesium, phosphorus, chromium, and molybdenum. The two minerals that we will talk about for their antioxidant activity are selenium and zinc.

About now you are saying, "Wait a minute. Aren't those metals? Do you mean iron like my grandma's skillet? And copper like the plumbing under my sink?" Basically, yes. Minerals are rocks and metals, but we are talking about having a few molecules of these minerals available to each cell in your body, not chunks of limestone or chrome plating on your kidneys. And you can't get the kind of minerals you need by swallowing iron filings. You can only absorb these minerals after they have been extracted from the earth by growing plants. They, in turn, process the minerals for you into an organic form that your body can use.

Chromium

[See "Diabetes Mellitus," chapter 4]

Chromium and Insulin Levels

Chromium improves glucose tolerance and lowers insulin levels. It also improves the efficiency of insulin.

Chromium-Rich Foods

Chromium-rich foods include brewer's yeast, string beans, cucumbers, soy foods, onion, garlic, and green foods.

Copper

Although excessive levels of copper in the body can result in oxidant-related pathologies, an optimum level of copper is generally required to maintain antioxidant defense, and copper deficiency, which is common, increases oxidative stress. Copper deficiency is related to a deficiency in the copper superoxide dismutase (Cu SOD) antioxidant defense system, participating in the breaking of the free radical chain of events.

Copper Linked to Cardiovascular Health

Copper is also linked to cardiovascular health. A deficiency of copper results in oxidative damage in both the heart and liver. Data suggests that a weak antioxidant defense system in the heart is responsible for the high degree of oxidative damage in the copper-deficient heart.

Copper Protects Skin Cells Against Ultraviolet Radiation

When combined with selenium, copper protects skin cells against ultraviolet radiation.

Copper and Anemia

Anemia has been associated with both copper and selenium deficiencies.

Manganese: Manganese is a key mineral, and along with zinc and copper, it plays a most important role in the superoxide dismutase antioxidant enzyme systems.

Magnesium

What Does Magnesium Do?

Magnesium is a mineral that helps make white blood cells, which are very important for fighting infections and diseases. It also combines with red blood cells. It combines with calcium and phosphorus, assuring strong bones and teeth. It helps with the utilization of vitamins B and E, fats, calcium, and other minerals.

What Are Food Sources for Magnesium?

- rice
- sesame
- soybeans
- kelp, dulse
- almonds, cashews
- raw/cooked leafy greens
- figs
- apples

Recommended dosage for magnesium is 750 to 1,000 milligrams.

Potassium

What Potassium Deficiency Does to Your Body

Potassium deficiency produces certain symptoms. Low body potassium is linked to low tissue oxygenation. Water accumulation is common, indicating difficulty in the kidneys. A common symptom is edema (swelling) of the ankles, which is a positive indicator of low tissue oxidation. The brain functions poorly with low potassium. The cerebellum is particularly affected. A person's physical movements become difficult and his balance uncertain. Mental work becomes difficult. Headache may be a common symptom. With a lack of potassium, the peristaltic activity of the bowel is defective. This may result in hyperacidity, the so-called "heartburn syndrome." In fact, hyperacidity of the entire body is related to hypopotassemia. "Additional signs of potassium deficiency include dry skin, skin eruptions, memory impairment, constipation, depression, diminished reflex activity, nervousness, at times insatiable thirst, fluctuations and arrhythmias of the heartbeat, high cholesterol, insomnia, low blood pressure, muscular fatigue and weakness."[47]

Finally, potassium is an essential mineral in the function of the adrenal gland, an important antistress endocrine organ. It is an integral part of the antistress system.

Sources of Potassium

Sources for potassium are primarily in the greens, the vegetables, and the cereals. Unfortunately, the cereals that are consumed primarily in our society lack the exterior component of the grain, and most of the potassium and other important substances are milled away, resulting in a cereal that is primarily starch. Supplemental potassium is, of course, available.

". . . [f]ood sources of potassium include dairy foods, fish, fruit, legumes, meat, poultry, vegetables and whole grains. Specifically, it is found in apricots, avocados, bananas, blackstrap molasses, brewer's yeast, brown rice, dates, dulse, figs, dried fruit, garlic, nuts, potatoes, raisins, winter squash, torulae, wheat bran, and yams."[48]

"Herbs which contain potassium include: catnip, hops, horse tail, nettle, plantain, red clover, sage, and skull cap."[49]

Selenium

What Is Selenium and Where Is it Found?

Selenium is a metal you may not have heard much about. It occurs all over the world, but in very small quantities, and it is usually combined with other metals. It is seen as a pollution threat, not because it is toxic, but because it likes to combine with sulfur to make all kinds of nasty stuff. It is not used much where you can see it, but selenium is in lots of things that you use around the house. For instance, do you have a transformer that converts alternating current (from your wall plug) to direct current (maybe for your youngster's Nintendo game or a cordless phone)? Inside that little box is a selenium circuit that does the job. It has unique abilities to transform energy from one form to another. It is used in solar energy panels because it can convert sunlight directly into electricity! For that same reason, it is used in all kinds of photoelectric cells from light meters to electric eyes. Interestingly enough, if you look at a chemistry periodic table, you will find out that selenium is in the oxygen family of elements. It was only recognized by the Food and Drug Administration (FDA) as an essential trace element in 1990.

Benefits Derived from Selenium as an Antioxidant

The number one benefit derived from selenium as an antioxidant is that it is required for the production of the enzyme glutathione peroxidase. All that you need to know about glutathione peroxidase is in the "Enzymes" section of chapter 5, so I won't try to explain it all here. The important truth about this enzyme is that it stops the oxidation of fats, especially LDL cholesterol. That means there will be less stuff clogging arteries, less heart disease, less death. This is a good thing! Study after study has shown that where there is heart disease, there is not enough glutathione peroxidase; and there is not enough glutathione peroxidase because there is not enough selenium available to keep production up. Selenium supplements turn it all around. The results of an experiment by Dr. Aviram of the Rambam Medical Center in Haifa, Israel, released in January 1998, showed that selenium supplements caused about 33 percent more glutathione activity, which led to a 46 percent decrease in LDL oxidation. In other words, selenium cut the amount of cholesterol ready to form arteriosclerotic plaque by half! When there is enough selenium, glutathione does its job and the conditions that caused the cardiovascular disease can be reversed. Unfortunately, the damage done by a cardiovascular crisis cannot be reversed as easily, so do not wait for a problem to come up. If this was the only reason to use selenium, it would be more than enough to justify any cost for supplementation. Just by this one action, selenium can save your life.

But that is not the only thing selenium does for us. Working together with vitamin E, it strengthens our immune system and thyroid functions and keeps our heart, liver, and pancreas healthy. Add zinc into that combination, and it reduces an enlarged prostate. It has even been found to protect the livers of alcoholics from cirrhosis. Since it is highly concentrated in sperm cells, it can also be linked to fertility. You can get too much selenium, but the symptoms of selenium toxicity are easy to spot: brittle hair and nails, garlicky breath, metallic taste in the mouth, and hair loss, and the liver and kidneys may start having trouble, the skin turning jaundiced.

Normal Dosages

If this should happen, you should reduce the dosage. Doses of as much as 700 micrograms daily have proven safe, even for extended periods. A normal dosage should be 200 micrograms per day, and unless you are eating a couple of acres of parsley each day, you are not getting it from your diet.

Selenium and Its Ability to Fight Cancer

One of the surprises of selenium is its ability to fight cancer. Dr. Larry Clark and his colleagues at the University of Arizona formed an experiment to see if taking selenium helped prevent skin cancer. If you live in Arizona, that is really important. They followed over a thousand people for ten years to see if 200 mcg a day would prevent skin cancer in older people who had already had a bout with it. The test was a miserable failure; the incidence of skin cancer was just about the same as for those who did not take selenium. *However*, there was a 37 percent drop in the number of other life-threatening cancers and a 50 percent reduction in the number of deaths from cancer. In fact, there were 46 percent fewer cases of lung cancer, 67 percent fewer esophageal cancers, 62 percent fewer colon cancers, and a whopping 72 percent reduction of prostate cancers! Pretty good failure, huh?

Those findings were confirmed in November 1997 when the International Epidemiology Institute published the results of a twelve-year, thirty-thousand-person global trial of the effectiveness of vitamin and mineral supplements. They found a clear connection between the intake of selenium working with vitamin E to significantly reduce the risks of cancer and cancer-related deaths. Another study by the National Cancer Institute examined the effects of different antioxidant combinations on cancer rates in Linxian, China, an area noted for low intake of many nutrients and a high risk of cancer and stroke. One group was given vitamin A with zinc, another received B complex, a third received C with molybdenum, and the fourth group took beta-carotene, vitamin E, and selenium. At the end of five years, the fourth group (those taking beta-carotene, vitamin E, and selenium) was found to have 9 percent fewer deaths, 13 percent fewer cancers, and a marked reduction in the number of strokes. These antioxidants really work! They do prevent cancer and stroke!

Selenium and the HIV Virus

But perhaps the most significant research is the ongoing studies into the relationship between selenium and the HIV virus. Ethan Will Taylor, M.D., a pathologist at the University of Georgia, has pioneered much of this research, and he cites these facts about selenium and AIDS.

- Selenium is required for proper immune system function, particularly the T-cells, the lymphocytes intimately linked to the scenario of Acquired Immunodeficiency Syndrome (AIDS).
- Selenium amplifies the action of interleukin-2 (IL-2), a natural immune system stimulator that has shown promise as a treatment for AIDS.
- There is a progressive decline of selenium levels in Human

Immunodeficiency virus (HIV) patients. This is a significant predictor of survival since decline of selenium parallels the progress of the disease. Some have noted that the
selenium levels are *surprisingly low in the early stages of
the disease* as well.

- Simple selenium compounds inhibit HIV growth in a test
  tube.

- "An immense body of evidence demonstrates the role of
  oxidative stress in stimulating HIV replication, that certain
  antioxidants can inhibit this process, and suggests the presence of an antioxidant defect in HIV patients."[50]

These facts led Dr. Taylor to hypothesize that perhaps the
declining selenium levels, rather than being a result of the disease,
were intimately connected with its cause. There are other viruses
that seem to only cause disease where there is a selenium deficiency, such as the hepatitis-B virus. Perhaps HIV is another one.
He suggests two mechanisms that could be at play here. One is
simply that decreased selenium means greater oxidative stress
because glutathione peroxidase levels are down (we are back to
that again). This could trigger growth of the virus or at least remove the inhibiting factor that was seen in the test tube with
selenium. The second mechanism is more complicated.

Dr. Taylor, hoping to discover whatever he could about the
genetic material in HIV, found something very interesting. There
is an "open gene" in the HIV virus, one that is waiting to be
matched up and completed by another amino acid (remember
that genes are amino acid chains) and that the amino acid it is
waiting for is UGA, the code for selenocysteine. This amino acid
form of selenium is not abundant in the body, but the immune
system uses it regularly and the body will form it as needed as
long as there is selenium present to do it. Not only is the virus
waiting for this selenoprotein, but this gene is in the middle of a
pattern that activates with glutathione peroxidase. To oversim-
plify the theory, it looks like the virus enters the body looking for
selenium. If it finds some, it plugs it into this gene and it is satis-
fied. It won't replicate! Selenium, like a switch, turns off the reproduction of the virus. But if there is even one virus cell that
does not get the selenium it wants, it starts reproducing itself and

the disease progresses accordingly. This certainly explains why selenium levels are low at the beginning of the disease; it has been used up trying to satisfy the virus! It may also explain why some people live with the HIV virus for years without showing any sign of the disease. They must have enough selenium to keep it in check. It also helps to explain why AIDS is more active among peoples who have poor nutrition (Haitians, Africans, intravenous drug users) and why the symptoms of selenium deficiency and AIDS look so strikingly similar.

For the present, this is all still theory. It may take a while to find all the answers and it may take even longer to convince the medical community that selenium plays a major role in the solution of AIDS. In the meantime, Dr. Richard Passwater noted in an interview at the Linus Pauling Institute: "All of the long-term HIV-positive survivors were taking selenium and NAC, as well as generous amounts of other antioxidant nutrients."[51]

Where Is Selenium Found?

Dietary selenium can be found in meats, fish, and a variety of grains. It is also found in brewer's yeast, broccoli, kelp, onions, and molasses. There is also a long list of herbs that contain selenium, including alfalfa, parsley, garlic, ginseng, and hawthorn berry.

Sulfur

[See "Garlic" chapter 5]

Where Is Sulfur Found and What Can It Do for Me?

Sulfur-containing foods, such as garlic, onions, leeks, scallions, chives, and shallots, are powerful antioxidants. Stephen L. DeFelice, M.D., the man who created the term "neutraceuticals," believes garlic, because of its enormous sulfur content, can stop cancer. A research study done at Memorial Sloan-Kettering Cancer Center in New York exposed fresh human prostate cancer cells to S-allymercaptocysteine (SAMC), a sulfur compound that is created when garlic ages, noted that the cancer cell growth diminished two to four times more quickly than normal.[52] Kyolic is the best garlic (aged garlic extract).

Important Cancer-Fighting Sulfur Compounds

Important sulfur compounds that help the body fight cancer are:

- Indoles—cancer-blocking agents
- Isothiocyanates—blocks and suppresses cancerous cells
- Thiols—sulfur-containing nutrients
- Cysteine—sulfur-containing amino acid
- Glutathione—sulfur-containing amino acid

Sulfur Food Sources

Sulfur food sources:

- eggs
- grains, wheat germ, granola, oatmeal
- vegetables—alfalfa, asparagus, broccoli, Brussels sprouts, cabbage, cauliflower, horseradish, mustard greens
- fruits—figs, plantain, ripe papaya, pineapple
- nuts/seeds—almonds, cashews, picons
- legumes—chickpeas, lentils

Sulfur Prevents Caramelization of Your Blood

Sulfur in the system prevents glycation (caramelization) of the blood. Just like when you caramelize sugar on the stove, your body caramelizes fats and sugars that you have eaten by its own internal heat source. So, our blood becomes darker and "syrupy," which gums up our cells biochemically. It's really important to eat these sulfur-containing foods as often as possible!

Zinc

What Is There to Know About Zinc?

Zinc? You've probably noticed that some multivitamins and cough drops have started advertising "with zinc" on the labels. One commercial even had a picture of a shower head showering your throat with zinc, a pretty strange image considering that zinc is metal. But why? What is it that we are all supposed to know about zinc that would make us want their products?

There is a lot to know about zinc. It has all kinds of different functions all over your body. Most important for our discussion is that it is the basis of over two hundred enzymes, including superoxide dismutase (SOD) and those enzymes responsible for the production of DNA and RNA. It also has a place in the structure of cell walls and the links that hold specific genes together in the DNA molecule. Those links are called "zinc fingers." Admittedly, they sound like the name of a comic book villain, when in fact they are vital in our genetics.

Among zinc's nonantioxidant roles, it boosts the immune system at the cellular level and increases the number of T-lymphocytes, which fight infection. It is essential for all cell growth and accelerates the healing of wounds. Even gastric ulcers can be healed by zinc. As an anti-inflammatory, it is helpful in controlling acne and arthritis. I have discovered that zinc helps the psoriasis victim. It is required for the senses of taste, smell, and vision and plays a big role in the development and function of male sexual organs and prostate. It also enhances the action of some hair-growth serums, but zinc by itself will not grow hair.

Zinc levels tend to fall off as we age, which leads us to believe that it is related to various problems associated with aging. For one thing, the decline in zinc levels parallels the decline in the immune system that corresponds with aging. That in itself could explain why many maladies afflict the elderly but ignore the young. It also opens the door for tissue degeneration, as damaged tissues are unable to count on zinc's healing powers.

Zinc and the Common Cold

As far as the cold cures, zinc has been found to shorten the time it takes to get over a cold. If you start taking zinc lozenges every two hours when you first start having symptoms, you can be finished with that cold in about four days instead of eight to ten days. A couple of studies did not get these results, but there are at least three studies that confirm the same findings. Taking zinc in pills does not help; it is the action of soaking the throat with the lozenges—putting zinc on the infected tissues—that makes it work.

Zinc is known to kill the viruses that cause colds, but the healing that it brings directly to irritated tissues is more likely due to antioxidant actions.

Zinc, Cancer, and Other Problems

In relation to cancer, zinc has many interesting functions. Lower zinc levels have been found in patients with esophageal, bronchial, and prostate cancers. Adding zinc to the diets of various rodents has stopped chemically induced cancer from starting. Also, the copper/zinc form of SOD and other antioxidant enzymes are lower in the cells that cancer corrupts. It appears that the cancer targets these cells with less protection. All of this points to zinc as a preventative to cancer. But it has also been found that cancer growth is slower when we take zinc away! The reason for this is probably that zinc, being essential for DNA synthesis, is necessary for *all* cell growth, even malignant growth. Taking away the zinc from established cancer cells keeps them from reproducing their malignancy.

Macular degeneration is another disease associated with both oxidative damage and declining zinc levels, though the cause is not really known. Zinc supplementation is not a cure for macular degeneration, but taking it has been proven to slow the loss of vision significantly at twelve- and twenty-four-month checkups. The cure will probably be found when we combine all the different antioxidants that affect the eye together.

Many of the symptoms of Down's syndrome can be treated with zinc. It has been proven to boost their immune system by improving thyroid and white cell functions and increasing lymphocyte activity. It also improved their ability to repair DNA damaged by radiation. Growth retardation in DS may also be related to zinc deficiency. Of the twenty-two children given zinc supplements in one test, fifteen reached a higher percentile on the growth chart. Children with DS also have a problem with immature blood cells that cannot carry oxygen. Zinc supplementation helped to cause these cells to die so that the body could replace them with healthy cells.

Zinc has a lot to offer diabetics. It plays a vital role in the production of insulin, first when insulin is stored in the beta-cells of the pancreas as zinc crystals, and later when insulin is bound to liver and fat cells. It might also be noted that one way to create

Main Trace Minerals

Mineral	Main Symptom of Deficiency	Dietary Source	Proportion of total body weight (%)
Calcium	Rickets in children; osteoporosis in adults	Milk; butter; cheese, sardines; green leafy vegetables; citrus fruits	2.5
Chromium	Adult-onset diabetes	Brewer's yeast; black pepper; liver; wholemeal bread; beer	<0.01
Copper	Anemia; Menkes' syndrome	Green vegetables; fish; oysters; liver	<0.01
Fluorine	tooth decay; possibly osteoporosis	Fluoridated drinking water; seafood; tea	<0.01
Iodine	Goiter; cretinism in new-born children	Seafood; salt-water fish; seaweed; iodized salt; table salt	<0.01
Iron	Anemia	Liver; kidney; green leafy vegetables; egg yolk; dried fruit; potatoes; molasses	0.01
Magnesium	Irregular heartbeat; muscular weakness; Insomnia	Green leafy vegetables (eaten raw); nuts; whole grains	0.07
Manganese	Not known in humans	Legumes; cereals; green leafy vegetables; tea	<0.01
Molybdenum	Not known in humans	Legumes; cereals; liver; kidney; some dark-green vegetables	<0.01
Phosphorus	Muscular weakness; bone pain; loss of appetite	Meat; poultry; fish; eggs; dried beans and peas; milk products	1.1
Potassium	Irregular heartbeat; muscular weakness; fatigue; kidney and lung failure	Fresh vegetables; meat; orange juice; bananas; bran	0.10
Selenium	Not known in humans	Seafood; cereals; meat; egg yolk; garlic	<0.01
Sodium	Impaired acid-base balance in body fluids (very rare)	Table salt; other naturally occurring salts	0.10
Zinc	Impaired wound healing; loss of appetite; impaired sexual development	Meat; whole grains; legumes; oysters; milk	<0.01

Taken from *The Cambridge Factfinder* (Cambridge University Press, 1994), p. 133.

diabetes in rats is to deprive them of zinc. Once the disease is under way, zinc can relieve some of the complications of diabetes. It can reverse the trend toward poor healing of wounds and may help overcome diabetic vision loss. Many diabetics are told to go on high-fiber diets, which is good for controlling blood sugar but bad for absorbing zinc. Anyone on a high-fiber diet should be sure to use a zinc supplement.

For daily supplementation, taking zinc in a multivitamin-mineral supplement makes the most sense. Then it can help in the absorption of vitamins E and A. Good "multi" supplements usually have enough zinc. The RDA for zinc is 15 milligrams, but recommended dosages would be 15–30 milligrams for adults and 10 milligrams for children. Grains, brewer's yeast, wheat bran and germ, and seafood are generally better sources of zinc than vegetables.

Zinc Dosages and Deficiency

It is possible to take too much zinc, but that would mean 100 milligrams daily for an extended period of time. Doses of up to 150 milligrams can be tolerated for short periods. One of the effects of too much zinc is that copper will not be absorbed. That destroys the chances of making copper/zinc SOD, and the immune system starts weakening. A balance of ten units of zinc to one unit of copper should be maintained. Other symptoms of excessive zinc are nausea, vomiting, and gastric distress. It can also inhibit HDL cholesterol—the good one—so that LDL levels start to rise.

Zinc deficiency is marked by slow growth; poor appetite; slow-healing wounds; abnormalities of taste, smell, and sight; and white flecks in the fingernails. It might also cause mental lethargy and lack of sex-gland functioning.

Zinc Is an Essential Mineral: Zinc is an essential mineral that is in most tissues of the body. It impacts the entire hormonal system and all the glands, especially the prostate. Zinc helps the defenders of your immune system do their jobs. It is a proven immunity builder which helps boost killer T-cells, helper T-cells, and suppressor T-cells. The T-cells identify antigens and rush to kill infected or cancerous cells.

Food sources for zinc:

- Oysters 6 med. raw (9–77 mg)
- Beef Shanks 3½ oz (9–77 mg)

- Crab 3½ oz (4–8 mg)
- Wheat germ ¼ cup (4–8 mg)
- Pumpkin seed 1 oz (0–3 mg)
- Ready-to-eat cereals 1 oz (0–3 mg)[53]

Soy

Soy Isoflavone Extract: The isoflavones in the germ portion of soybeans have been proven to be beneficial in both fighting and preventing cancer. These natural substances, especially the isoflavones genistein and possibly daidzein, have phytoestrogenic and antioxidant qualities that play an important role in the anticancer effect of soygerm. In fact, genistein is given credit by some researchers for the lower rate of beast cancer in Asian women whose basic diet includes soy.

In a study of five human–breast cancer cell lines, genistein inhibited the growth of all five types of cancer cells. This finding has been corroborated in similar studies showing that genistein significantly inhibits breast cancer cells by affecting the estrogen receptors in a way that prevents breast cancer from developing.

What is Soy and Where does it Come From?

What is soy? "Soy"(sometimes "soya") is the name for various foods made from soy beans. Soy beans are related to clover, peas, and alfalfa. The beans are processed in various ways and usually are in the forms of soy sauce, soy drinks, and soy curds. Soy is one of the few plant foods that contains an essential and proper balance of amino acids. This fact makes soy a particularly good protein source. Soy is especially valuable because it is equally low in fat and high in fiber, excellent for maintaining a balanced and healthy diet.[54]

Soy's Isoflavone called "Genistein" Inhibits the Growth of Cancer Cells

"The isoflavone called genistein is soy's antioxidant star. Isoflavones are compounds found in soy that contribute to its antioxidant powers. Many studies have shown how effective isoflavones can be and one isoflavone turns out to be the real star."[55] This is genistein. Its only source is in soy. Innumerable studies and many papers have been done confirming the fact that genistein inhibits the growth of cancer cells.

Researchers Suspect that Genistein Blocked Cancer Growth in Japanese Men

Of interest to me personally is this quote from Earl Mindell: "It's a fact that autopsies of Japanese men show that prostate cancer is as common in Japan as it is in the U.S., but the cancer seems to grow much more slowly. So slowly, in fact, many men die without ever developing clinical disease. Researchers suspect that genistein is blocking the growth of these cancers."

Finnish Researchers' Conclusions as to the Benefits of Genistein

One Finnish researcher and his colleagues compared the levels of isoflavones in Japanese and Finnish men. The levels of the isoflavones were more than one hundred times higher among the Japanese, with genistein occurring in the highest concentration of any of the isoflavones. The researchers' conclusion, published in *Lancet*, was that "maintaining a lifelong concentration of isoflavones in the blood could be the reason why Japanese prostate cancers remain latent."[56]

U.S. Studies Show Genistein Blocks Breast Cancer Cell Growth

A University of Alabama study (1990) showed genistein reduced the number of tumors in breast cancer experiments in animals. The researchers at Alabama found that genistein not only blocks estrogen, but also blocks the breast cancer cell growth.

Soy Lowers Cholesterol and Helps in the Prevention of Heart Disease

Mindell continues, "[a]ll of these various studies and their results show that genistein, unique to soy, its fellow isoflavones, and other important components of soy, are very interesting characters in the unfolding story of cancer prevention and protection."[57]

Soy lowers cholesterol and helps prevent heart disease, according to Dr. Mindell.

He further states that a Japanese study published in the annals of the *New York Academy of Sciences* found that the oxidation of LDL "was greatly reduced in rabbits fed on soy milk."[58]

An Italian Study Also Found a Drop in Cholesterol Levels When Adding Soy to Diet

"A study in Milan, Italy, found a similar preventive effect in a group of volunteers who were all on low-fat diets and had high cholesterol levels. Those adding soy to their diets saw a drop in their cholesterol within just two weeks, while levels did not fall in those not eating soy. Even when cholesterol was deliberately added to their diets, soy eaters still experienced the same drop in cholesterol. *In fact, in Italy's nationalized health service, a soy protein is provided free of charge to doctors for the treatment of high cholesterol*" [emphasis added].[59]

Soy Is an Effective Cancer Blocker

Back to soy and cancer. Soy is an effective cancer blocker because of its isoflavone content. These isoflavones resemble the hormone estrogen and they occupy the estrogen receptor sites, but they do not behave like the estrogens, which, in excess and unopposed by progesterone, are known carcinogens. These isoflavones are "thousands of times weaker than the estrogens and actually act as anticancer compounds."[60] This is similar to the way tamoxifen, the most widely used drug in breast cancer therapy, works.

Studies in England revealed that isoflavones can be an effective treatment for premenopausal women with breast cancer and other cancers associated with estrogen.

Risk of Cancer Reduced by One Half for Those Who Eat Soy Frequently

A 1991 study reported in *Lancet* revealed that the risk of breast cancer in those who rarely ate soy foods was twice as high as for those who ate soy frequently.

A similar cancer comparison study was done in the United States by a Harvard researcher who found that Americans in South Dakota and Wyoming who regularly ate soy beans had less than half the risk of getting cancer of the colon as those who did not eat soy.

Soy and Menopause, Diabetes, Cataracts, and Kidney Damage

Dr. Mindell went on to state, "soy products reduce menopausal symptoms. Soy products lower the need for insulin in diabetes. Soy prevents cataracts. Soy is an excellent source of protein for the patient with kidney damage, being much easier to metabolize and excrete than protein derived from an animal source."[61]

Consumption of Soy: How to Get It into your Diet

According to Dr. Mindell, "Japanese men consume 40 to 70 milligrams of genistein per day. U.S. men eat less than one milligram."[62]

Further, he states, "[t]here are many ways to incorporate soy into your diet from soy protein powders to soy milk, miso soup, and tofu. Soy comes in many different forms, including soy milk, tofu, tempeh, miso, soy sauce, and soy flour. These are all made in varied ways, including fermentation, soaking, grinding, frying, steaming, and sprouting. It would appear that tempeh and tofu are the best ways to eat soy. Soy sauce contains the least amount of beneficial nutrients and is high in sodium."[63]

What Can Soy do for Me?

Here is what soy can do to help you. It will prevent heart disease. It will lower cholesterol (LDL). It will reduce menopausal symptoms, prevent many types of cancer, prevent cataracts, maintain healthy kidneys, reduce diabetic need for insulin, and help prevent osteoporosis in that soy consumption results in less calcium loss than does animal protein consumption.

A University of Texas study, using volunteers replacing animal products with soy products in their diets, saw a 50 percent drop in calcium loss in their urine.

Vitamins

Give Your Body the Nutrients It Needs

Now that we have discussed the problem of oxidative stress and the illnesses it can cause, let's talk about the solution. Amazingly enough, the dilemma of oxidation can be overcome. Your body has the built-in mechanisms necessary to not only neutralize free radicals (oxidants), but to heal the damage they cause. The solution lies in the way your body was originally designed to operate *if it is given the proper nutrients*! In particular, your body needs various substances called antioxidants because of their activity to fight oxidants and oxidation. To reiterate from previous chapters, oxidants are the free radical bad guys, and antioxidants are the proverbial heros that restore your body's balance and physical well-being.

According to Drs. Elaine Conner and Matthew Grisham,[64] the following are some "naturally occurring antioxidants": albumin, ascorbic acid, bilirubin, carotenoids, sulphydryl groups, a-tocopherol, Co-Q-10 (Ubiquinol 10), and uric acid. There are many others, and many as yet unidentified. Synthetic antioxidants include: acetylcysteine, glutathione esters, nitroxides, penacillamine, probucol, and tamoxifen. Another way of dividing antioxidants would by those produced by your body and those that must be taken in through diet and supplements. Honestly, there are many substances of all types that play different roles in fighting oxidation, and we are only beginning to learn about how they work. Each one seems to work just a little differently from all the others, so they have to be discussed individually. Not only that, they have unique and amazing ways of working together, which are just now coming to light.

Sources of Antioxidants

I feel that it is vital that you know about the four main sources of antioxidant chemicals (enzymes, herbs, minerals, and vitamins), as well as other major subareas (amino acids, bioflavonoids, and carotenoids), and individual antioxidants which are equally of great importance (Co-Q-10, DHEA, green foods, green tea, and soy). By discussing the various groups identified, I am hoping to hit the most important of these chemicals and give you an idea of how the antioxidant system in your body works.

Vitamins in General

Vitamins are considered micronutrients in that they are needed in relatively small amounts, compared to the amounts of proteins, carbohydrates, and fats our bodies need. They assist in regulating metabolism and releasing the energy from digested food. They also act as coenzymes, catalysts that activate enzyme activity. While you may not need huge quantities of them, vitamins are essential to health because they work at the cellular level, which is where the real battle for health is fought.

Vitamins are divided between those soluble in water and those soluble in oil (fat). Vitamins A, D, E, and K are considered oil (fat) soluble. As such, they can be stored in fat for some time and toxic levels of these vitamins can be built up if taken in massive doses for a period of time. Vitamins B and C are carried through the body in water and any excess is carried away and discarded daily. This means that they must be replenished daily. The vitamins that have special antioxidant properties are A, B, C, E, and P. Vitamin P is a relatively recently discovered set of substances called bioflavonoids.

Vitamin A

As one of the fat-soluble vitamins, vitamin A is crucial in maintaining the health of moist, soft tissues such as mucous membranes, skin, hair, and eyes. If there is a deficiency of vitamin A, it will show up first as dryness of these areas. It may also manifest itself as infections of these tissues like acne, sinusitis, and respiratory infections and may go on to include stunted growth, insomnia, fatigue, and weight loss. But vitamin A is also important to the development of bones and teeth. It aids in the storage of fat, and protein cannot be metabolized without it. Of course, vitamin A's claim to fame is that it is the reason your mother always told you, "Eat your carrots; they're good for your eyes." She was right. It enables better night vision, protects the moist tissues of the eye, and promotes normal vision.

Where Is Vitamin A Found?

Vitamin A is found in two basic forms, retinol and carotenoids. Retinol is also known as "preformed" vitamin A because it is the form found in animals, ready to do its work. Retinol is found primarily in animal food sources, such as cod liver oil, liver, egg yolks, and dairy products. Carotenoids, especially beta-carotene, are called "provitamin" in that they are converted into vitamin A by the liver. Carotenoids are found in plant food sources like dark green leafy vegetables (spinach, broccoli), yellow-orange vegetables (carrots, squash, cantaloupe, peaches), and red vegetables (tomatoes). The biggest difference between these two forms of vitamin A is that you can consume large quantities of beta-carotene without any side effects (well almost, your skin might turn a little yellow), but retinol, being a fat-soluble vitamin, can become toxic if taken in large doses over a period of time. Natural beta-carotene is always best. Other carotenoids include alpha- and gamma-carotene, lutein, and lycopene, but beta-carotene is the one most closely associated with vitamin A.

Since we have an extensive portion of this chapter devoted to the carotenoids, this present section will deal with retinol and vitamin A's work in the body.

What Does Vitamin A Do for My Body?

As an antioxidant, vitamin A has several important jobs, especially in protecting cell membranes and fatty tissues. Most important, it helps repair the damage done to mucous membranes by smoking and pollutants. This is something that affects everyone. Even nonsmokers are confronted with the fact that their respiratory tract and eye tissues are constantly assaulted by pollutants in the air. The free radical bad guys (oxidants) are rampant in these toxins, which cause oxidative damage, yet your most sensitive tissues are openly exposed to them. As a potent antioxidant, vitamin A neutralizes free radicals (oxidants), helps to repair any damage they have done, and if infection should set in, vitamin A is there to boost your immune system to counteract it. vitamin A does everything it can to keep these vital tissues healthy.

Vitamin A Particularly Important for Smokers

For those who smoke, vitamin A is an absolute must! The tissues of the mouth, sinuses, trachea, and lungs that you are scorching with each cigarette need lots of help to overcome the abuse you are inflicting on them. The same goes for everyone around you who has to breathe your smoke.

Vitamin A Also Boosts the Immune System

We mentioned boosting the immune system. This is another job of vitamin A. It helps to fight infections of the respiratory tissues and viral infections like cold and flu. One way that it does this is by enhancing the "germ receptors" on antibodies so that they are more likely to attack and not ignore foreign bodies. Researchers found that even moderate supplementation of carotenoids over a short period of time made a big difference in how monocytes (white blood cells) responded to infection. There is more about this study in the section on beta-carotene.

Another study showed that vitamin A supplements changed the type of immune response. Normally, when exposed to the Newcastle virus, chickens would produce a T-helper white blood cell type response, but after a diet high in vitamin A, they produced a more aggressive T-cell and more antigens were produced both at the cellular and tissue levels. In other words, they fought the infection harder and more efficiently.

Vitamin A and Radiation

Another problem that affects everyone is radiation, but vitamin A can help here, too. A group of rats faced whole-body X-ray radiation and were then checked for DNA damage in their bone marrow and in their white blood cell count. Those who had been on a vitamin A–rich diet showed significantly less DNA mutations and much higher leukocyte levels. They also had about four times as much vitamin A stored in their livers as the mice who were irradiated on a normal diet. This indicates that radiation eats up vitamin A because it increases the need to fight free radicals and that having enough retinol available reduces the damage that radiation can do to your DNA and your immune system.

Vitamin A and Colitis

Oxidative damage to the mucous membrane of the intestines is key to the progression of ulcerative colitis. A 1997 study in Vellore, India, has shown that patients with active colitis have plasma levels of vitamin A and cysteine, both important antioxidants, that are sharply lower than those in healthy individuals and that they grow lower as the disease becomes more severe. It was discovered also that these levels returned to normal within two weeks after the disease has been treated. While they have not yet studied specific treatments, these researchers suggest that intervening to correct this deficiency of vitamin A and cysteine at the early stages of the disease may be a way to halt its progression by minimizing oxidative damage.

Vitamin A and Various Forms of Cancer

Various forms of cancer can be prevented by vitamin A also. By increasing the sensitivity of the immune system, retinol wakes up the tumor-surveillance monitors so that cancers can be fought. By protecting DNA within body cells, vitamin A reduces the harmful mutations caused by radiation that can lead to cancer.

Best Food Sources for Vitamin A:

- Alfalfa
- Apricots
- Beets
- Broccoli
- Cantaloupe
- Carrot
- Dandelion greens
- Garlic
- Kale
- Mustard
- Papaya
- Parsley
- Peaches
- Pumpkins
- Spinach
- Sweet potatoes
- Swiss chard
- Turnip greens
- Watercress
- Yellow squash

A diet rich in vitamin A vegetables provides both fiber and antioxidant protection to reduce the risk of colon cancer, according to a study at the University of Montreal. While the Southwest Skin Cancer Prevention Study Group could not see a benefit in vitamin A supplements for patients at high risk who had already had melanomas, they did show that supplements can reduce the chance of a first cancer ever appearing for people at moderate risk. The incidence of breast cancer is related both to the intake of fruits and vegetables containing vitamin A and to the amount of vitamin A and carotenoids stored in the adipose tissues of the breast. Finally, the M. D. Anderson Cancer Center in Houston has found that retinol and compounds related to it actually help in the process of gene transcription—that is, the copying of genes when a new cell is formed. If there is enough vitamin A, the genes copy more accurately and that means fewer cancers get started. Their research is particularly impressive because they were studying second cancers in people who had already been treated for cancer of the head, neck, and lung areas. Since these are the tissues most likely to be affected by smoking and pollution, this study suggests that even after cancer has appeared once, a second cancer can be avoided with vitamin A supplementation.

Vitamin A (Retinol) and Diabetes

Retinol has a strange relationship to diabetes that is not fully understood yet. One thing that is clear is that retinol is required for insulin release. Islet of Langerhans cells in the pancreas, when flooded with retinol, produced twice as much insulin as those depleted of vitamin A (*Pancreas*, July 1997). But there seems to be a problem getting the vitamin where it needs to go in the diabetic. When supplements were given to induced-diabetic rats, the amount of vitamin A in the bloodstream remained low, while the amount in the liver increased. This problem of not being able to transfer vitamin A where it is needed is probably why blindness is a common outcome of long-term diabetes. The nutrient simply never makes it from the liver to the retina, leading to slow degeneration of the sight organ. It appears that vitamin A is not transported because of decreased availability of its carrier proteins, but it is not known why this happens. Simple supplementation is probably not the answer here, since that could lead to a toxic overload of the liver, but further research could find that solving this problem may lead to breakthroughs of all kinds in treating diabetes.

Vitamin A, Smoking, Atherosclerosis, and Cardiovascular Disease

A French study took a group of smokers and a gro up of non-smokers and changed their diet. Both groups were made to eat enough fruits and vegetables to supply 30 milligrams of carotenoids a day for two weeks. The researchers found that the carotenoids circulating in the participants' blood increased by 23 percent in the smokers and 11 percent in the nonsmokers. At the same time, the participants' resistance to LDL oxidation (a key step in the formation of arterial plaque and hardening of the arteries) increased by 14 percent in the smokers and 28 percent in the nonsmokers. This was a modest change in their diet for only a short period of time, but it had a big effect on their health and reduced their risk of atherosclerosis.[65] Another way that vitamin A fights cardiovascular disease is that it promotes healthy endothelial cells, which line the inside of blood vessels. By fighting oxidation of this thin layer of tissue, it also protects the smooth muscle cells below it from becoming rigid and unresponsive. It is important that the smooth muscle cells maintain their ability to contract and keep pushing the blood along.

A healthy endothelium also prevents oxidized LDL from attaching to the arterial wall, forming plaque and ultimately blockage. There is an Italian study that showed a significantly reduced risk of heart attack in women who ate diets high in beta-carotene, but the same study did not associate consumption of retinol with any reduced risk. So vitamin A keeps your arteries healthy, stops LDL oxidation, and reduces your risk of heart attack. What more could you ask for?

Vitamin A and Recommended Dosages

Vitamin A seems to be most effective with adequate levels of protein (10–20 percent of total calories from protein) and zinc (15 milligrams per day). The optimum levels for taking vitamin A in the form of retinol would be about 5,000–25,000 I.U. per day for adults. ("I.U." means "international units.") Half that amount is fine for teenagers, and only 2,000–3,000 I.U.s per day is needed for children. But don't forget that there are a multitude of benefits from eating the fruits and vegetables that contain the provitamin carotenoids, so seek these foods out first, then supplement. Vitamin A's effectiveness is diminished by use of mineral oil and the lack of vitamin D in the body.

The B Vitamins

Folic Acid and Pantothenic Acid

There is a group of related chemicals that we have lumped together as B vitamins. They can be taken individually, but they are usually found in B complex supplements, which contain most, if not all, of the eleven chemicals. They are primarily thought of as membrane stabilizers and natural tranquilizers. The B vitamins are not generally known as antioxidants, but there have been a few recent studies that indicate a significant antioxidant effect for at least two of the B vitamins: folic acid and pantothenic acid.

Some of the earliest studies came from the Nencki Institute of Experimental Biology in Warsaw, Poland, in late 1995 and 1996. Their studies of Ehrlich ascites tumor cells revealed several surprises about pantothenic acid. Their first conclusion was that pantothenic acid protects the cells from lipid peroxidation. Then they found that the mitochondria are also protected, even when samples are irradiated with ultraviolet light. While pantothenic acid was not observed scavenging free radicals itself, it was clearly the cause of elevated levels of glutathione (a protein that repairs hydrogen peroxide's damage to cell walls) and Co-enzyme A, which we have already discussed as a fat-cell repairer. In this way, pantothenic acid supplementation becomes the means to fight this form of cancer through antioxidant activity.

Folic acid is known mostly for its importance as a prenatal vitamin that reduces birth defects. It is now drawing a lot of attention as an antioxidant and more particularly as a cancer fighter. It is being used in conjunction with other agents as a part of chemotherapy in cancers of the entire digestive tract: aerodigestive, gastric, and colon cancers. In a study published in January 1998, chemotherapy that included folic acid was pumped straight into the artery that feeds the liver for a solid twenty-four-hour period once a week for twelve weeks. These were patients whose disease was advanced enough that the cancer was spreading from the colon to the liver and was too big to cut out. The results were impressive. Almost half of the patients either went into partial remission or stabilization of the disease. Fifty-fifty odds may not sound that great to you, but with a cancer this advanced, that's pretty good for the current state of medicine. Another study a few months earlier had about the same results when looking at the colon cancer alone. A third study, from September 1997, showed that this method worked even better in cases where part of the liver could be resected (tumor removed and tissue reconnected). That research showed that recurrence was delayed from an average of seventeen months to sixty-three months. That adds another three to five years to the lives of these people who really had almost no chance before. Best of all, the side effects for this type of chemotherapy are mild, with only a third of the patients suffering from nausea or vomiting, and it can be done in an outpatient setting.

How Does Folic Acid Help in the Treatment of Colon Cancer?

The reason folic acid works in the treatment of colon cancer is that it undoes the damage done to the DNA and RNA by oxidation. It works as a coenzyme to make sure that the genetic material in each cell replicates properly, eliminating the mutations that lead to cancerous growths. Gerard Bleiberg's conclusion (*Rev. Med. Bruxelles*, Sept. 1997) shows how important this discovery is: "For patients with disseminated disease, 5FU/FA [*the FA is folic acid*] based treatments allows a doubling in survival as compared to the best supportive care. Moreover, quality of life is significantly improved."

Folic Acid and Ovarian Cancers

An Italian research team has shown that reduced folate carrier (RFC) is a controlling factor in the progress of ovarian cancers. Notice, that was reduced folate, which means folic acid that has neutralized a free radical and needs repair. When the enzyme that carries these injured warriors to be patched up is inhibited, there is a 70 percent drop in the amount of folic acid in the cell. That means there must be a lot of folic acid working on oxidized particles, trying to correct the cancerous condition.

Folic Acid and Pancreatic Cancer

Pancreatic cancer is one of the most certainly fatal of all cancers, and it tends to spread to other organs very quickly. In order to find some kind of help for these patients, doctors at the University of Ulm, Germany, tried a combination of drugs in chemotherapy with both resected and nonresected cancer patients. The major constituent of the therapy was folic acid. They found that this treatment had amazingly little toxicity (less than 6 percent of those treated) and stretched survival times from three to five months to four to twelve months, and in some cases twenty-one months! That is not the same as complete recovery, but it is valuable and precious time for those patients and their families. And it is a move in the right direction. More research in this direction may find the right antioxidants to reverse the cancer completely.

Folic Acid and High Cholesterol Counts, High Levels of Homocysteine

But cancer is not the only condition affected by folic acid. It has also been associated with healing oxidative damage to endothelial cells that line the blood vessels. In patients with high cholesterol counts, a form of folic acid (5-methyltetrahydrofolate) was found to reverse the constriction of blood vessels and restore nitric oxide activity, which stops the oxidation of LDL cholesterol. Another study found that B vitamin supplements (folic acid, B_{12}, and B_6) given for six months, reduced homocysteine from 12.8 to 3.5 mumol/L. Still another study, seeking to find a reason for heart disease in diabetes patients, concluded that high levels of homocysteine were caused, in part, by inadequate folic acid availability. Bottom line: not having enough folic acid increased the risk of cardiovascular disease and heart attack, but supplementing folic acid *reversed* some of the key symptoms of the disease.

Folic Acid and Arthritis

Folic acid has also been identified as one of the nutrients in which people with rheumatoid arthritis are deficient. The other nutrients on the list? They are the standard antioxidants: vitamin E, calcium, zinc, and selenium. Apparently, it is the antioxidant quality of folic acid that is lacking in 54 percent of the people who develop arthritis. Also, patients treated with methotrexate had a significantly lower intake of folic acid than those on other therapies and should be aware of this so that they can adjust their diet.

While the exact mechanics of antioxidant activity for folic acid has not yet been mapped out, the effects that it has in each of these treatments shows a strong correlation to the way other antioxidants work in these same diseases.

B Complex and Recommended Dosages

A dose of 100 milligrams of B complex (B100s) is normally suggested, taken one to three times a day with meals. If taken on an empty stomach, expect some stomach discomfort and nausea. Being water-soluble vitamins, they are not stored in the body, and any excess will simply be eliminated. Normally, when you take B complex, your urine will be a bright yellow and have a pungent odor. This is evidence that your body really has absorbed the riboflavonoids in the vitamin and everything is fine. In fact, if you take a B complex vitamin and you don't have this happen, your body didn't get the nutrients, and you should switch to a brand that is more bioavailable. Women using oral contraceptives and people under stress use more B vitamins and should adjust their supplements accordingly.

Best Food Sources for B vitamins:

- Alfalfa
- Asparagus
- Brewer's yeast
- Brown rice
- Brussels sprouts
- Buckwheat flour
- Egg yolk
- Fresh peas (legumes)
- Kidney beans
- Lentils
- Lima beans
- Nuts
- Oats
- Seeds
- Soy products
- Wheat germ
- Whole grains

Recommended dose: 100 to 300 mg per day. Best taken with meals.

Vitamin C

Historical Notes on the Discovery of Vitamin C

An English naval doctor was given the task of finding a solution to the problem of scurvy in the ranks of Her Majesty's fleet. Dr. Lind found that simply feeding these men citrus fruits, oranges, and lemons cured the disease and prevented it from occurring in others. That was in 1747. Fifty-three years later, in 1800, the British Royal Navy finally took his advice seriously and introduced lemon juice into the diet of shipboard seamen. The incidence of scurvy dropped from 1,457 cases in 1780 to only two cases in 1806. But it was not until 1928 that Noble laureate Albert Szent-Gyorgi isolated the chemical responsible for these dramatic results, and it became known as vitamin C, ascorbic acid. Then, in the early 1960s, Dr. Jonas Salk, already noted for his discovery of the polio vaccine, became a proponent of vitamin C for fighting the common cold. In the mind of the common man, this raised the activity of this vitamin from superstition to medicine, even though there were two hundred years of research to prove its effectiveness.

Today the problem is not in convincing people that vitamin C works, but in trying to find out just how many different things it can do. It seems to be everywhere and do everything. Since it is vital in the formation of collagen, it plays a role in tissue growth and repair, including healing and healthy gums. It also keeps teeth and bones strong. The immune system is enhanced by vitamin C, and it helps in the production of certain hormones.

How to Get Vitamin C Into Your Body

The body does not manufacture vitamin C at all, so it must be taken in through diet and supplements. Since it is a water-soluble vitamin, there is no threat of overdose, but high doses taken orally are usually eliminated through the urine. Moderate doses taken several times a day would give better results, but if you really need high doses, it is best to take it intravenously, under a doctor's supervision. It is also best to take estified C (Ester-C), which is created by linking ascorbic acid with a dietary mineral like calcium, potassium, or zinc. This form of vitamin C is nonacidic and is absorbed by the body much better. By the way, chewable vitamin C is hard on your teeth. Don't use it.

Vitamin C Combats the Effects of Water and Air Pollution

As an antioxidant, vitamin C should be considered a foundational part of your antioxidant supplementation. One of its greatest benefits is that it fights the effects of pollution. As we take in pollutants in the air we breathe and the water we drink, all of that toxicity produces free radicals. Vitamin C does wonders to neutralize these radicals. Smokers, who pollute their air on purpose, are especially prone to have lower vitamin C levels because of the simple fact that their reserves are eaten up with each cigarette. This leaves the smoker's immune system weakened and depletes his or her antioxidant capability, thereby opening him or her up to the possibility of cancer, cardiovascular disease, and other sickness.

Vitamin C and Cardiovascular Disease

Vitamin C also helps fight cardiovascular disease. By protecting the endothelium (the lining of the artery) from oxidative damage, it promotes better blood flow, even in patients with high blood pressure. A study in the journal *Circulation* (Nov. 1997) demonstrated that vitamin C reduced the number of superoxide radicals in the arteries, and thereby reduced the number of LDL particles that oxidized. Simply by reducing the number of free radicals floating around, vitamin C has an indirect effect on stopping lipid peroxidation, which leads to atherosclerosis.

Vitamin C and Diabetes

Diabetics tend to have problems with vitamin C because this nutrient likes to ride on insulin to be carried through the body. So diabetics tend to have low vitamin C levels simply because there is not enough insulin to circulate it. This means that diabetics also have problems with not having enough antioxidant activity, at least the ones who do not take insulin. Dr. S. R. Maxwell et al., showed that this lack of antioxidant activity results in poor control of the diabetes. So the antioxidants don't circulate when insulin is low and then the insulin level tends to crash because there are not enough antioxidants. It is a vicious circle that leads to more rapid progression of the diabetes. Being aware of this and supplementing vitamin C may slow that progress. Likewise, attacks of acute hypoglycemia (low blood sugar) cause a rush of free radicals, which use up the available antioxidants and bring on oxidative stress.

Wide swings, either high or low, result in excessive free radical activity. Therefore, antioxidants are a must if you continue to indulge in refined sugar and other sweets.

Vitamin C and Lung Cancer, Prostate Cancer

Various kinds of cancer have also been associated with vitamin C. A study of more than ten thousand men and women surveyed and followed up with nineteen years later showed that vitamin C intake played a crucial role in preventing lung cancer, with the risk being 66 percent greater for those who consumed the least ascorbate. A new study involving prostate cancer suggests that ascorbic acid inhibits the division and growth of cancerous cells. This means it can be used to treat cancer as well as prevent it.

Vitamin C and Cataracts, Lens Opacities

Researchers were aware that vitamin C helped reduce cataracts, but new evidence has established that connection in a remarkable way. The *American Journal of Clinical Nutrition* reports that women age fifty-six to seventy-one who had used vitamin C supplements for ten years or more had a 77 percent lower incidence of lens opacities. If we looked at moderate lens opacity, there were

83 percent fewer cases. The key in this study was the long-term use of supplements, which gave long-term protection and turned back the clock to reverse the effects of aging.

How Vitamin C Works

It has been mentioned before that one of the key parts of the cell that oxidation will strike is the mitochondria, the energy generators for the cell. Mitochondria have elaborate defenses against oxidation, but one of the key factors in keeping the mitochondria healthy is to not let them be attacked in the first place. This is where vitamin C comes in. Floating in the liquid of the cell, vitamin C can neutralize free radicals before they ever reach the membrane of the mitochondria. This reduces the amount of energy it takes for the mitochondria to fight oxidation and leaves more energy for the life of the cell. This is particularly important because we now know (*Molecular Cell Biology*, Sept. 1997) that as long as the mitochondria maintain a high energy level, they will win the fight against oxidation. So vitamin C especially plays a vital role in conserving that energy.

One of the most fascinating features of how vitamin C works is the way it interacts with other antioxidants. A study at Tufts University has shown that taking just 220 milligrams of vitamin C boosts the levels of vitamin E by 18 percent and raises beta-carotene levels by 13 percent. Apparently vitamin C regenerates the other nutrients after they have been used to neutralize free radicals. Several studies have demonstrated that when vitamin E reacts with an oxidative particle, it becomes a vitamin E radical, having lost one of its electrons. Vitamin C comes along and restores that vitamin E back to its original state, so it can be recycled and used again. Only in October 1997 was it observed that vitamin E can return the favor and regenerate vitamin C as well. Normally, vitamin C will keep on regenerating vitamin E until all of the ascorbic acid is depleted, and only then will vitamin E start dwindling. If you keep a steady intake of vitamin C, that should never happen. In this way, the water-soluble antioxidants and the fat-soluble ones work together, producing synergistic effects that are much greater than any one nutrient working alone.

Best Food Sources for Vitamin C:

- Asparagus
- Avocados
- Beet greens
- Broccoli
- Brussels sprouts
- Cantaloupes
- Collards
- Currants
- Grapefruit
- Green peas
- Kale
- Lemons
- Mangoes
- Mustard greens
- Onions
- Oranges
- Papaya
- Parsley
- Persimmons
- Pineapple
- Radishes
- Rose hips
- Spinach
- Strawberries
- Sweet peppers
- Swiss chard
- Tomatoes
- Turnip greens
- Turnips
- Watercress

Recommended dose: 1,000 to 5,000 mg in divided dosages daily.

Vitamin E

Tocopherols, Tocotrienols, and d-Alpha Tocopherol

Vitamin E was first recognized by the Food and Nutrition Board in 1968 as an essential vitamin. By definition, it is essential because the body cannot manufacture its own vitamin E and therefore it must be provided by foods and/or supplements. As an oil-soluble vitamin, excess vitamin E is not eliminated from the body immediately but is stored in fat for several days. Vitamin E is not a single compound, but a group of eight slightly different chemicals divided into two major groups called tocopherols and tocotrienols. The most important and effective of these is called d-alpha tocopherol.

What Are the Important Things Vitamin E Does For My Body?

Aside from its antioxidant properties, vitamin E is recognized as being important in healing, repairing damaged tissues, and reducing scars. It also lowers blood pressure, helps prevent anemia, and supports normal clotting. It is associated with healthy nerves, muscle, skin, and hair. Other effects range from aiding premenstrual syndrome to relaxing leg cramps to preventing cataracts.

Natural Vitamin E versus Synthetic Vitamin E— "d-alpha tocopherol" Is the Most Effective!

Natural vitamin E and synthetic vitamin E are not equivalent. According to *The Vitamin E Fact Book*, natural-source vitamin E is isolated from vegetable oils, whereas synthetic vitamin E is produced from petrochemicals. Natural-source vitamin E is delineated as "d-alpha tocopherol," a single entity; whereas synthetic vitamin E, "dl-alpha-tocopherol," is a mixture of eight isomers, only one of which is molecularly equivalent to natural vitamin E. Studies in both humans and animals indicate that natural vitamin E (or d-alpha tocopherol) is nearly twice as effective as synthetic vitamin E.

Vitamin E and Heart Disease, Atherosclerosis

Vitamin E is one of the most versatile antioxidants. It has been linked to most of the degenerative diseases we have discussed, most notably heart disease. In atherosclerosis, according to Dr. Malcom Mitchinson, "[t]he diseased human artery has been found to contain oxidized fats; antioxidants diminish the development of atherosclerosis in experimental animals; and there is evidence from human population studies that high antioxidant intake protects against the complications of atherosclerosis. Vitamin E supplements offer real hope of eradicating this dreadful disease."

In an interview in *Whole Foods* magazine ("How Vitamin E Prevents Heart Disease"), researcher Dr. David Janero explains this process in more detail. He explains that modified or damaged low density lipoprotein (LDL) tends to set off certain "scavenger receptors" on the surface of macrophages (antibodies) in the blood vessel, so that the macrophages internalize the LDL. This creates bloated macrophage cells, known as foam cells, which tend to line the wall of the vessel and build up to form plaque. Plaque creates a hazard in three ways: 1) it narrows the passageway of the vessel, leading to blockage; 2) it hardens the vessel wall so that it cannot assist the blood flow; and 3) pieces of plaque can break off and embolize (float in the bloodstream), potentially lodging in and causing blockages in the smaller vessels of the heart, lungs, brain, and other organs. Since atherosclerosis is most likely to affect the coronary and carotid arteries, which supply blood to the heart muscle and brain respectively, the danger of embolism is particularly severe.

Dr. Janero also speaks of a second factor in atherosclerosis, the corruption of the normally smooth muscle cells in the vascular wall. In order for the foam cells to find a place to stick in the blood vessel, there must be some disruption of the endothelium, the lining of the arterial wall. One of the key contributors to damage in the endothelial cells is lipid peroxidation. With exposure to oxidants (free radicals—ROS), arachidonic acid is released from the cell membranes of the arterial lining. The cell membrane's lipids are thus converted to toxic peroxides. In turn, this damages the membrane's ability to assimilate nutrients and increases cellular mutation. This creates just enough damage for the foam cells to stick and begin the formation of plaque. In the *Whole Foods* article, Dr. Janero states:

> Vitamin E is a critical antioxidant protector of endothelial-cell membranes against the consequences of oxidative stress, particularly lipid peroxidation. More limited data suggest that vitamin E can promote endothelial repair and even suppress harmful oxidant production within the endothelium itself, which could lead to, for instance, oxidation of lipoproteins.

How Vitamin E Fights Atherosclerosis

To put vitamin E research into more understandable terms, here are five specific ways in which the experimental evidence shows how vitamin E is able to fight blockage and eventual heart disease:

1. Vitamin E inhibits oxidation of lipoproteins in the blood vessels.
2. Plaque lesions caused by long-term deficiency of vitamin E can be limited, if not reversed, with usage of vitamin E.
3. Vitamin E supplementation reduces the incidence of atherosclerosis.
4. Vitamin E helps improve blood-lipid profiles, reducing triglycerides and LDL cholesterol, which are most likely to oxidize and be trapped by macrophages.
5. In population studies, there is a correlation between higher vitamin E levels and reduced deaths from heart disease.

Plaque in Your Arteries + Abnormal Clotting = Obstruction (Heart Attack or Stroke)

Another complication of oxidants (free radicals—ROS) in the bloodstream is that platelets, when oxidized, produce thromboxane, which results in abnormal clot formation. Arterial plaque plus abnormal clotting leads to arterial obstruction, causing heart attack and stroke. Vitamin E and other antioxidants can prevent this scenario from developing.

Vitamin E and Heavy Eating

A vascular benefit of vitamin E is in reducing the vascular stress caused by heavy eating. Normally, when a person eats a high-fat meal, there is a serious decrease in blood vessel function for the next two to four hours. In other words, blood flow is decreased, which explains the lethargic feeling we have after eating a heavy meal. A study reported in the *Journal of the American Medical Association* (*JAMA* 278 (1997), pp. 1682–1686) showed that when vitamin E and C were taken before that heavy meal, that problem was prevented. "The end result with the vitamins was comparable to that of the low-fat meal."

This is truly important information! Before you head to Wendy's or the Dairy Queen, take some vitamin C and E.

Vitamin E and Recommended Dosages

The dosage required to make a significant difference in coronary health may be considerably higher than you might expect. The RDA (recommended daily allowance) for vitamin E is only 30 I.U.s per day, which is enough to sustain life but not even close to the amount required to promote health. One study, using healthy subjects, recommended a dosage of 500 I.U.s per day to significantly reduce LDL susceptibility to oxidation. In this study, results were achieved in six weeks. In another study, testing patients with cardiovascular disease, the dosage had to be increased to 800 I.U.s per day, administered with 1,000 milligrams of vitamin C and 24 milligrams of beta-carotene, and results were not seen until the twelfth week. This would indicate that we need considerably more vitamin E than we think we do (up to 250 times more!) and that we need even more than that if a problem has already developed.

On the other hand, a study of elderly patients published in the *Journal of the American College of Nutrition* (August 1997) suggested that even low dosages can still be beneficial. With very low doses of about half of the recommended daily allowance of various vitamins and minerals, antioxidant activity still increased after about six months. By the end of the two-year study, there were consistent increases of up to four times the ability to handle oxidation. The most important thing this study teaches us is that *consistency* of antioxidant intake is more important than quantity. I recommend a dosage range of 400 to 1,200 I.U.s daily.

Long-Term Use of Antioxidants Is Recommended

To have any real effect upon atherosclerosis and cardiovascular health, *long-term* use of antioxidants is required. This is not a "quick fix," but part of a lifestyle change: a commitment, with a perseverant attitude toward safeguarding and enhancing your cardiovascular system.

Vitamin E Works in Synergy with Other Antioxidants

While vitamin E is a potent antioxidant by itself, its effects are magnified when it works in harmony (synergy) with other antioxidants. In the case of coronary health, selenium is found to work with vitamin E to prevent cardiomyopathy, and vitamin C boosts the level of vitamin E found in the blood. A Japanese study recently explained this relationship. It found that high dosages of vitamin E alone produced an oxidative tocopherol radical, which counteracted the effects of taking vitamin E, but that when vitamins E and C were taken together, the C vitamin reduced the tocopherol radical back to vitamin E, making it usable as an antioxidant again.

One source of a nearly perfect combination of antioxidants for heart health in a whole food is vine-grown tomatoes. They contain vitamins C and E, along with the carotenoids beta-carotene and lycopene. Dr. Aviram of the Rambam Medical Center in Israel has shown that pure tomato extract (as in the product Lyc-O-Mato™) dramatically increases the resistance of LDL cholesterol to oxidation. The reason for its effectiveness is the combination of anti-oxidants working in a complementary and supportive way to increase overall antioxidant capability.

Vitamin E and Aging

In relation to aging, *Health* magazine listed vitamin E discoveries as one of the top ten medical advances for 1997: "In the never-ending quest for an anti-aging pill, Vitamin E emerged as a leading candidate in 1997." A study at Tufts University showed that vitamin E's immune system enhancement results in increased resistance to infection and pneumonia, common problems of the elderly. At doses of just 200 milligrams a day, subjects showed two to six times the disease-fighting ability of the control group.

Vitamin E and Increased Cognitive Abilities

Another recent study tested the cognitive abilities of 260 people from age sixty-five to ninety, then analyzed their diets and correlated nutrition to their scores. The results showed that diets high in antioxidant intake yielded higher test scores. So did diets low in fat and high in carbohydrates. In short, thinking ability and memory were better in those elderly people who gave their bodies the right nutrition *regardless of their age.*

Vitamin E and Parkinson's Disease

A population study in Rotterdam, the Netherlands, concluded that there was a definite link between the intake of vitamin E and Parkinson's disease. While the study did not seek to use vitamin E as a treatment for the disorder, it did establish a dose-dependent relationship between the intake of vitamin E and the occurrence of Parkinson's disease. They concluded that "a high dietary intake of vitamin E may protect against the occurrence of [Parkinson's disease]."

Vitamin E and Alzheimer's Disease

The most astounding finding of the year was in vitamin E's effect on Alzheimer's disease. A nationwide study, the largest ever, tracked the progress of 341 patients diagnosed with Alzheimer's in fairly advanced stages. For the first time ever, a medication was found that slowed the progression of the disease: vitamin E. Four milestones were indicated in the progress of the disease: the onset of severe dementia, loss of ability to perform simple tasks, institutionalization, and death. Vitamin E postponed the patients' reaching each of these milestones by two hundred days or more. That means prolonging their enjoyment of life by seven months at each stage. A synthetic drug, selegiline, showed almost identical effects. "The rationale is that these drugs could interfere with the process of brain-cell death. Oxidizing agents are formed as a result of the progressive brain cell death in Alzheimer's disease, and they themselves are very toxic to brain cells. We hoped that vitamin E and selegiline might interfere with that process." Why wasn't this discovered before? Probably because the dosage given in this study was 2,000 I.U.s per day, which is more than sixty times the recommended allowance! Earlier researchers would not have attempted to use such a high dosage because they did not understand how antioxidants worked.

The following chart will help you see how much vitamin E you are taking in and find some other sources that you might want to try.

TYPICAL VITAMIN E CONTENT OF SELECTED FOODS
(Based on alpha-tocopherol content)

Food (100g portion)	I.U. of Vitamin E	Food (100g portion)	I.U. of Vitamin E
Oils and Fats		Bread, white	0.21
Wheat germ oil	177.97	Corn flakes, cereal	0.16
Sunflower oil	72.56	White rice, boiled	0.13
Safflower oil	58.97		
Peanut oil	28.13		
Margarine, soft	20.66	**Nuts**	
Mayonnaise	19.32	Sunflower seeds, raw	73.76
Margarine, hard	16.01	Almonds	40.53
Soybean oil	11.80	Peanuts, dry roasted	10.73
Butter	3.22	Peanut butter	9.24
		Cashews	0.28
Grains			
Oatmeal, rolled, cereal	2.02	**Meat, fish, eggs, milk**	
Brown rice, boiled	2.01	Liver, broiled	0.94
Bread, whole wheat	0.80	Shrimp, frozen, baked	0.89

Food (100g portion)	I.U. of Vitamin E	Food (100g portion)	I.U. of Vitamin E
Chicken, fried	0.86	Bananas, fresh	0.33
Eggs	0.69	Cantaloupe, fresh	0.21
Bacon	0.67	Strawberries, fresh	0.19
Haddock	0.64		
Chicken breast, broiled	0.55	**Vegetables**	
Steak, broiled	0.45	Spinach, fresh	2.67
Whole milk	0.06	Peas, fresh	0.82
		Broccoli, fresh	0.69
Fruits		Beans, Boston baked	0.21
Apples, fresh	0.46	Potato, baked	0.05

Calculations based on: J. B. Bauernfeind, "Tocopherols in Foods." In *Vitamin E: A Comprehensive Treatise* (1980): 133–155.

Best Food Sources for Vitamin E

- All green-leafy vegetables
- Brown rice
- Cold-pressed oils
- Cornmeal
- Dry beans
- Eggs
- Milk
- Nuts
- Oatmeal
- Wheat germ

Recommended dose: 400 to 1,200 I.U.s daily.

Vitamin E Reduces Heart Attack Risk: The Cambridge Heart Antioxidant Study was a controlled trial conducted in England at the Clinical School at Cambridge University and at the Papworth Hospital, where two thousand heart-disease patients participated. Half of these patients were prescribed high-dose vitamin E (400–800 I.U.s daily) and the other half were given a placebo. After eighteen months, vitamin E was determined to have reduced documented heart attacks by a striking 75 percent. This particular study was published in the March 23, 1996, issue of the *Lancet*.

According to Dr. Morris Brown, a lead researcher in the study, "We are enormously excited to discover that vitamin E really is as beneficial as we had all hoped. *Now we can confidently say that Vitamin E protected against heart attacks*" [emphasis added].

Taken from an article in "The Health Store News" (October 1997): "Vitamin E Reduces Heart Attack Risk," by Karen Kleiner.

Vitamin P (Bioflavonoids)

Where Is Vitamin P Found?

In 1936, vitamin pioneer Albert Szent-Gyorgyi was performing experiments to see why vitamin C extracted from lemons was more effective than pure ascorbic acid. He found a substance in the white rind of citrus fruits that seemed to have a beneficial effect on the strength of capillaries, yet still let oxygen, carbon dioxide, and nutrients pass through the capillary walls. He named it vitamin P because it affected capillary permeability. Later on, it was found in the pulp of citrus fruits and many vegetables as well. As research continued, it became clear that this was not a single chemical, but a collection of substances with similar structures. So far we have found about three thousand different nutrients that we lump together in this family.

In 1950, the American Institute of Nutrition examined the evidence available and decided that this family of chemicals should be considered "pharmacological agents" rather than vitamins. In their thinking, a vitamin is something that, if you take it away, has a specific set of deficiency symptoms. That is why their recommendations are always based on what you need to keep from getting sick. Since they could not find any specific deficiency syndrome for vitamin P, they decided it didn't classify as a vitamin and, since there were so many different substances, suggested the name "bioflavonoids." We also call them flavonoids for short. Since there are no "non-bio-" flavonoids—they all come from living plants—the name "bioflavonoids" is repetitively redundant all over again.

The Twelve Groups of Flavonoids

To simplify things, the flavonoids can be broken up into twelve groups based on chemical structure: anthocyanins, anthocyanidins, leucoanthocyanins, flavones, flavonols, flavonones, flavonolols, isoflavones, chalcones, dihydrochalcones, aurones, and catechins. Now, to simplify the simplification, there are a whole bunch of chemicals with little variations. Each group is characterized by specific antioxidant actions and the foods that produce them. For instance, *anthocyanins* are found primarily in berries and grapes, and their primary benefit is to fight cancer by protecting the cells' DNA from free radical damage.

- *Flavones* have the same benefit as anthocyanins but are found in green vegetables like celery and parsley.
- *Flavonols* can be further divided into:
  - *catechins*—which are found in tea;
  - *kaempferol*—found in endive, grapefruit, leeks, and radishes; and
  - *quercetin*—which comes from apple skins, broccoli, olive oil, onions, oranges, red wine, and tomatoes.
- The flavonols are associated with lowering cholesterol and reducing the risk of heart disease. Some of them also combat cancer.
- *Flavonones* are the flavonoids (say that three times fast) that Szent-Gyorgyi found in the rind of citrus fruit. Grapefruit rind has the most and its number one job is to fight infection.
- *Isoflavones* are different. They come from soy bean products and they have an effect on the female hormones. They stop the spread of estrogen-dependent cancers and they can alleviate menopause symptoms.

Bioflavonoids Make the Red and Blue Colors in Plants

What all bioflavonoids have in common is that they make the red and blue colors we see in plants. (The orange and yellow colors are caused by carotenoids.) Also, they all have a hydroxyl group somewhere in their structure. Guess what a hydroxyl group is good for? That's right! It eats up hydroxyl radicals and other free radicals. Some flavonoids are so good at stopping hydrogen peroxide from oxidizing fats that they are being equated to BHT, the preservative that food manufacturers put in potato chips, margarine, and ice cream to make sure the fats in those foods do not go bad. In plants, their contribution to the color of the plant plays a role in pollination, but they also fight microbes and fungi that could infect the plant. When we eat them, we do not get much benefit from the color, but we do benefit from their antimicrobial and antifungal qualities.

Pycnogenol Is Very Powerful

Some flavonoids are more powerful than others, but generally it is the combination of several different flavonoids that make them effective. That is the case with Pycnogenol. It is not a single chemical, but a combination of about forty different bioflavonoids all working together and in different ways that makes this supplement so effective. In fact, bioflavonoids are probably the real workhorses behind every herbal remedy. For instance, bilberries contain anthocyanidins known to fight infection. Milk thistle extract contains silymarin, which is used to treat liver disease. Rutin is a flavonoid linked with sugar that is thought to be the effective component in ginkgo biloba.

Bioflavonoids Have Side Benefits

Bioflavonoids have side benefits that come from their antioxidant activity. In addition to reducing the number of free radicals we are carrying around, flavonoids also chelate metals in the body so that they do not generate more radicals. Another side effect is that flavonoids stabilize collagen. You may be thinking that only affects the people who have their lips injected with it, but your body uses collagen to rebuild tendons, cartilage, and muscle all over your body. Flavonoids also inhibit certain enzymes that are involved in stimulating viral replication, cataracts, and asthma and allergy responses. Plus, one of the by-products of their infection-fighting activity becomes the basis for Co-Enzyme Q-10, which does a plethora of good things for you.

Antibacterial Bacteria? One of the more fascinating aspects of flavonoids is that only about half of what you take into your body is directly absorbed into the bloodstream. The rest is broken down by the bacteria normally found in the GI tract. Some of the by-products of this process are organic acids that contribute greatly to the body's ability to fight off unwanted bacteria. So the good bacteria in your digestive system produce the chemicals that fight the bad bacteria found in infections.

Which Bioflavonoids Do You Need?

All of them, of course. That is why a diet that consists mainly of fruits and vegetables is so important. But also be aware that cooking can destroy many of the flavonoids, as well as the vitamins in foods, so eating live foods is also a good idea. The three flavonoids that are found in most supplements are hesperidin, rutin, and quercetin. Each of these is important, but anthocyanidins and catechins are just as important. Look for a supplement that has as wide a range of flavonoids as possible. Some companies put flavonoid compounds in with herbs and vitamins that have complementary functions. The RDA has set no minimum requirement for bioflavonoids, and there has not been any toxicity seen at higher levels, so the amount you take is pretty wide open. Normally, a person on a wholesome, balanced diet probably consumes about 1,000 milligrams a day, so supplementation of around 500 milligrams is reasonable.

CHAPTER SIX

Integration of the Whole

The Whole

"Being whole" is the key to better health. The needs of each bodily cell must be met, with nothing lacking, for health to be possible. Here, we are not so much concerned with the health of individual cells; instead, we are concerned with the health of a person, the *whole* person. Unless the body, mind, and soul of this whole person are all healthy, no one considers him truly healthy. If this premise is correct and true health is a result of this "whole person" concept. Therefore, it is vital that we address and understand the optimal functioning of this "whole person" to achieve freedom from both physical and mental diseases. This means that we must look beyond the body as a machine, recognizing the important immaterial aspects of man as well. At times, these nontangible, nonmechanical aspects of humanity form the environment in which the body thrives. It is my belief that one of the body's roles is to serve the higher endeavors of mankind, our spiritual oneness, yet the corporeal and ethereal are so intrinsically linked in us that they are impossible to separate. Doctors are beginning to understand that emotional health may be more important to physical health than any virus, cholesterol level, carcinogen, or other disease-causing mechanism.

Wholeness might be defined as health restored, the needs of the whole person being met. Here the internal environments of the body and mind are stabilized and in perfect balance. This is balance at all levels, from the whole to each system, to each organ, to each cell, to each chemical reaction within each cell. It is particularly these smallest levels that affect us most, for when the cells do not work properly, the organ malfunctions. Many of the reasons for problems at the chemical level have to do with lifestyle choices that the whole person makes and lives out. Even the choice between a positive or negative attitude about life sets up a set of chemical alterations in the brain that affect the whole body. All effective remedies for disease must take into consideration the whole person: mind, body, soul. Restoration of the body's health (wholeness) begins with an understanding that supplying the body with "good things" is foundational to becoming this whole person.

Good Things for the Body

Wholeness must begin with providing the body with all that it needs to maintain its proper balance and function. This means we must maintain a balance of activity and rest, of heat and cold, of fat and lean; for any extreme of these things leads to imbalance and sickness. Imbalance leads to stress, as some other part must compensate for the part that is out of balance. Unresolved stress kills, and the only way to alleviate this stress is to give the affected parts of the body all the nutrients that they need, first to heal, then to function normally.

Try this: Stand on one foot. Notice that the foot you are standing on suddenly becomes much more active, pushing against the ground in a variety of ways to maintain your balance. Now lean forward as far as you can without falling. Do you feel the stress in your foot and your calf? Maybe even in your thigh and hip? You can sit down now. That leg was having to compensate for the fact that the other leg was not doing its job. It had to do things that it was not used to doing, not really strong enough to do, and could not keep doing for an extended period of time, and there was probably some degree of pain involved. In order to reduce the pain, you had to remove the stress, give that leg a chance to relax, and let the blood come back in to wash out the stress toxins and bring in nourishment.

No matter what kind of imbalance we put ourselves through, the same kind of thing happens. If your heart is not beating strongly, the blood vessels try to compensate, and your blood pressure goes up. If one eye is weak, the other tries to compensate and stresses itself until it becomes weak as well. If you stay cold for a long time, your body compensates by putting all of its energy toward keeping you warm, but the immune system is soon weakened and you catch a cold. If you fail to get the rest you need, that creates stress. *All imbalances create stress!* You can handle stress when it is a temporary situation, but chronic and/or long-term imbalances take a real toll on all of us. We have to find a way to relieve the stress, give that part a chance to rest, and give it all that it needs to heal.

So what good things does the body need? Throughout this book you've found many recommendations, but generally what the body needs are four basic things to acheive wholeness: water, food, exercise, and rest. We will address the added components of the soul and spirit in a moment.

Good Things for the Body — Water

About two thirds of your body's weight is water. It is the main component of every cell in your body except bone, and it is absolutely essential for the life of every cell in your body. Almost everything your body does requires water, too. It takes water to create energy. It takes water to burn fat. It takes water to chew and digest food. It takes water to heal wounds. It takes water to think, to breathe, and to make blood for muscles to move. Everything your body does takes water. Your body can go for weeks without food, but only a few days without water. By the way, the one and only substance that can get fat out of our bodies is water. Take your bodyweight and divide by two. Drink that many ounces of water each day for a month, eat normally, and see what happens to your weight. It may be the easiest diet you'll ever find.

Unfortunately, most of us don't take our bodies' need for water seriously and fail to drink anything close to the eight 8-ounce glasses of water a day that our bodies require. Coffee doesn't count, and neither do soft drinks, tea, juices, or beer. You need pure water to flush out all the junk those other drinks left behind. Water is also one of our primary sources of oxygen, which sustains life, as we talked about in previous chapters. Note: Consider OxyWater™ oxidized water. It may be the best available on the market today.

The second challenge is that most of the water available to us is poison. Municipal water supplies treat water as if they cannot afford to purify it. Even if they did, the contamination in the plumbing from the treatment plant to your tap would undo what they had done. (Have you ever seen what is inside the pipes in your house?) Much of the bottled water that is sold commercially comes straight from those same municipal water supplies. Those bottled waters which do, in fact, come from special springs may not be necessarily pure. There is no telling what toxins are in the ground near that spring and/or what contaminants were picked up in the bottling process. The only way to know what you are getting is to filter your own water using a high-quality filter. Even most of the filters you find in the stores do little more than remove the taste of chlorine from the water. Do the research for yourself to see what system is best for you. The National Sanitation Foundation (www.nsf.org) is a non-profit, independent testing agency that rates most of the leading filters and tells you exactly what they will filter out. Expect to spend several hundred dollars for a reverse-osmosis or quality carbon block filtration system. Sounds expensive, but that still works out to be less than half the cost of bottled water over the course of a year and much less in subsequent years when your only expense is to replace the filter.

Food

There are three different balances that have to be maintained in regard to food: 1) balancing the number of calories coming in with the number of calories being burned; 2) balancing protein, carbohydrates, and fat; and 3) balancing all the nutrients that your body needs. Just because you eat twenty-five hundred calories a day does not mean that you have gotten all the nutrients you need, and chances are you ate too much fat to get there. We are not going to turn this into a diet book. There are plenty of books that tell you what you should eat and which constituents are in which foods. We'll make it simple. Eat as many live fresh foods as you can. "Eat color" is a good suggestion. Eat as many green, yellow, orange, and red foods as you can. Don't eat processed foods. That is pretty much what we have said over and over again throughout the book. Amazingly, if you eat foods that have good nutritional value, you tend to have about the right balance of lean and fat in your diet as well and you are less likely to take in too many calories.

Counting calories can be a real drag, unless you are a really compulsive person. We can also kid ourselves into thinking that the size of the serving of cheesecake in the calorie counter bears some resemblance to the slab of cheesecake we just put on our plate. Rather than playing those games, try some easy-to-live-by rules.

1. Eat in moderation. If you eat until you are stuffed, that is too many calories, guaranteed. Leave the table hungry.
2. Eat regularly. Starving yourself makes your body think there is a famine, so it stores fat.
3. Eat 4 to 5 small meals a day. It keeps your metabolism burning faster.
4. Try to keep fat to about 30 percent of your calorie intake, not 30 percent of the food on your plate! Fat contains 9 calories per gram. Everything else contains 4 calories per gram, carbohydrates and proteins alike. So fat should only be about 10 to 15 percent of the weight of the food on your plate, and that has to include the fat cooked into your food. Pay really close attention to your fat intake for one month and then stay with the good habits that you have developed, and you won't have to count calories ever again.

Nutritional balance has been the subject of the whole book, so only a few comments need to be made here. The soil in which we grow our food has been abused greatly over the last two centuries and has not been replenished, so the food we buy does not have the same nutritional content it did even fifty years ago. We also have developed artificial maturity for many of these foods, such as green tomatoes and oranges sprayed with carotenoids to make them appear ripe when they reach the supermarket shelves. The fact is that they do not have the same nutritional value as vine-ripened fruits. The problem of pesticides has not gone away, either. Yes, we need to eat well and try to get as much nutrition as we can from a variety of fresh foods, but it is not likely that we will get all that we need in that way. For most of us, that means supplementation because our diets simply cannot give us all that we need. Think of vitamin supplements as a cheap insurance policy against the variety of diseases that are caused by not having the nutrients you need.

Processed foods are another problem. By definition, the nutrients have been processed right out of them. Counterfeit foods, those created by man, are unable to supply what the body needs to maintain stability and wholeness. Wholeness cannot be attained from them. Don't be deceived. Although processed foods look good and taste good, they are lacking in nutritional value and often contain toxic substances that damage and destroy your internal environment. The food God made contains the essential nutrients, enzymes, bioflavonoids, and carotenoids that are necessary to maintain the body's healing force within. Without them the body perishes before its time. It is sad, but true, that people are perishing because they do not know.

Exercise

Exercise is something we all know about, so there is no need to belabor the point. But most people don't exercise at all because they think it won't do any good unless they run a marathon each week. The fact is that it doesn't take much exercise to make a big difference in your quality of life. You don't have to run; you can walk. Walking is actually better for general health purposes. You don't have to do it for two hours. Twenty to thirty minutes is enough. The idea is just to elevate your heart rate for about twenty minutes. You don't have to do it every day. Three times a week will bring great reward.

What will it do for you? It will make your heart work just a little harder so that it stays strong. It increases blood flow to all those spots that forgot what blood felt like. It flushes toxins out of muscles that you haven't used in a while. It makes the lymph move in your lymphatics, cleansing and healing them. Mostly, it increases the amount of oxygen you are breathing in and circulating in your blood. That brings about the positive oxygen metabolism that fights free radicals and avoids the negative nitrogen metabolism where free radicals like to grow.

Also, you don't have to do aerobic exercise to get aerobic benefits. Anaerobic exercise should not be equated to anaerobic metabolism. You do breathe when you lift weights (*i.e.*, aerobic exercise). Research has shown over and over again that moderate weight training with a proper diet can strengthen the heart, slow the heart rate, lower blood pressure, increase lung capacity, and cause weight loss. A well-paced workout with weights (meaning you don't take a five-minute break between sets) two to three times a week will actually burn more calories over the course of the week than running a half hour four times a week. The reason is simple: when you stop running, the muscles stop asking for more food, but when you do five sets of leg presses, the same muscles crave food for the next two to three days while they rebuild and your metabolism increases. One of my assistants swears he can lose five pounds in a week just by adding three sets of deadlifts to his routine on Monday.

The bottom line is not what kind of exercise you do, but that you do something. Go play tennis. Go walk around the mall. Go chop wood. I like to play golf. Just go do something! The best exercise is the one that you will do because you like to do it and know it is "a good thing." It doesn't even have to look like exercise as long as there is a consistent activity level for about twenty to thirty minutes three times a week. The difference it will make in the way you feel will astound you.

Rest

The final ingredient for the health of the body is rest, which you will need after you exercise. Rest is the time when your body rebuilds what you tore down all day long. It is also the time when your brain sorts all the information it gathered that day and files it away for future reference. Without rest, your body feels weak and your brain gets confused. Eventually, your breath becomes shallow, your heart is stressed, and you are reverting to that anaerobic metabolism that free radicals love to live in.

The National Sleep Foundation says that Americans are "woefully ignorant" about the amount of sleep they need. We keep hearing stories about how Winston Churchill only slept four hours a night and Margaret Thatcher only five. We think we ought to be able to do the same. But we don't hear about Albert Einstein so often. He slept ten hours a night. Was he less successful? While 98 percent of us think that sleep is as important to health as nutrition and exercise, 64 percent of us get less than eight hours of sleep a night and half of those sleep less than six hours. So what is keeping us up? Finding a cure for cancer? Solving world hunger? How about television and the Internet. We just can't seem to turn it off. We've got to see one more late-night rerun of *Star Trek* or follow just one more computer link. All of a sudden it's 2:00 A.M. and you have to be up at 6:00 A.M. Then we wonder why our melatonin levels are messed up. That is bad enough if we are talking about older people, who are notorious for insomnia, but the primary offenders today are people in their teens and twenties. Maybe they need to rethink all that espresso they are drinking.

There is no shame in getting enough sleep. It is highly likely that you will be more productive in your waking hours if you get more sleep. That might alleviate the feeling of tiredness and frustration that keeps you looking for fulfillment in that extra hour of television. There is an even greater danger in that all of these sleepy people are driving around town. About one hundred thousand accidents a year are caused by drivers who have fallen asleep, resulting in fifteen hundred deaths and seventy-one thousand injuries. So get some sleep; the life you save may be your own.

Good Things for the Soul

Along with the physical stresses we encounter, there are also emotional stresses. Emotional problems put just as much stress on the body as physical factors do, and often more! Notice that it is the *body* that takes the burden of *emotional* stress. Why is that?

Man is not simply a machine. He is not just a physical mechanism. It is clear that there is an ethereal part to man, just as most religions have taught for centuries and medicine has acknowledged with the advancement of psychology (literally, *"the study of the soul"*). This noncorporeal aspect houses the mind (which transcends the brain, as Sir John Eccles demonstrated), the emotions, the will, memories, and desire. None of these functions can be assigned to any specific organ, yet they are what make us truly human.

The function of the soul, especially the emotions, is to provide an interface between the body and the wholly nonmaterial parts of man (his mind and will). As such, emotions are both a physical and an attitudinal response. Though we think of emotions as happening in our mind, we feel them in our body. When we feel fear, our pulse quickens and there is a very real adrenaline rush. When we are angry, the muscles of our neck and face tighten and we have a tremendous surge of energy that must be released. Sadness is felt more in our torso, as if our heart is heavy. It is no wonder that the ancient Hebrews considered the bowels to be the seat of the emotions.

Remember that these are called E-motions, energy motions. They are energetic responses that our body makes, and they demand to be physically acted out. Unfortunately, emotional expression is socially unacceptable for some, and others are simply afraid of what might come out if they allowed themselves to feel. Whatever the reason, many of us keep our emotions locked up, meaning that we keep all of that energy locked up, too. We repress (push back) instead of express (push out). All of that energy is trapped in our bodies, and it eventually starts acting out in whatever way it can on our internal parts. Ulcers, colitis, sinus problems, muscle tension, asthma, and sexual dysfunction are commonly found to have psychosomatic causes. More extreme cases result in hysterical blindness or paralysis. The energy is real and it will act on something. Since it takes less energy to let the emotion out than to keep it in, we need to find acceptable and safe ways to express our emotions. It is the best thing we can do for our health.

That is not just opinion; it is now accepted as medical fact. Dr. Dean Ornish recently published a book called *Love and Survival: The Scientific Basis for the Healing Power of Intimacy* (HarperCollins, 1998). In it, he cites study after study showing that emotional health and connection to others plays a *greater* role in maintaining physical health and healing than *any* medical intervention. He says, "I am not aware of any other factor in medicine—not diet, not smoking, not genetics, not drugs, not surgery—that has a greater impact on our quality of life, incidence of illness, and premature death from all causes." Dr. Ornish is noted for his treatment of heart patients using weekly support groups and lifestyle changes. You can read his book to learn all of the details, but here is a synopsis of a few of the studies he describes:

- Healthy men who responded "my wife does not love me" were three times more likely to develop an ulcer within the next five years.

- 95 percent of college students expressing negative views of their parents were found to have been diagnosed with a serious disease by midlife.

- Those who are socially isolated have a risk two to five times greater of premature death from all causes than those who feel a close sense of connection and community.

- 50 percent of unmarried men die within five years after clearing a blocked artery. This was three times the death rate among married men in the group.

- After open-heart surgery, those not participating in a regular social activity were four times more likely to die within six months. Those taking no comfort from religious faith were three times more likely to die in the same time frame. Those with neither social affiliation or religious hope were seven times more likely to die.

- Women with terminally advanced breast cancer were put in a support group for one year while a control group did not participate. At the end of five years, those in the support group had lived, on average, twice as long as those without a support group, some of them still surviving. All of the control group had died.

Dr. Ornish comments that if there were a drug developed by a pharmaceutical company that had these same kinds of results, there would be a media frenzy and every M.D. in the country would be prescribing it by the truckload. But when was the last time you heard of a doctor prescribing a regular dose of love and intimacy?

To maintain health, we must learn to nourish our soul and give it all that it needs to stay in balance. No one can live an emotionless life, and it wouldn't be much of a life if we could. But we can learn to communicate our feelings with others and to balance negative emotions with positive ones.

Here are some simple suggestions:

Limit the time spent in worry. Set aside an hour or so each week for concentrated worry. Then go enjoy your life the rest of the week. Worry is unproductive, causes physical stress, and is one of the most selfish behaviors there is. Most of what you worry about will never come to pass, the rest you can't control. If it is something you do something about, quit worrying and go do it.

Cultivate friendships with people who support and uplift you. And you can do the same for them. Social, business, and charitable organizations where everyone is working toward a single purpose may be helpful in meeting people. However, the best type of group support comes from a setting in which feelings and experiences can be shared without fear of judgment from any member. The intimacy developed in these groups and the relationship skills learned equip us with both transparency and boundaries in all of our relationships.

Receive and give ten significant touches each day. A misguided experiment was done in the seventeenth century to determine which language children would speak if not influenced by their caregivers. The children were left in their beds with no physical contact, even when fed. None of the children survived to the age when they might speak. Touch is important. The largest organ of your body is not your liver, but your skin, and its primary purpose is the sense of touch. Touch helps us to feel connected and loved.

It has been found that the critical number of touches we need to feel good about ourselves is ten. That doesn't mean ten people that bump you on the elevator; it is ten significant touches. Touch that has meaning. Hugs, kisses, and snuggles are clearly significant and if you can find ten of those, great. Other touches are just as important: a pat on the back, a squeeze on the arm, stroking of the hair or face, even a high five. All of these tell you that you are appreciated, you have value, you are precious. Handshakes don't really count, because that has become a formality, but you can add a significant hand on the shoulder or a two-handed shake to give it extra meaning.

What if you are not getting ten significant touches a day? The best way to get them is to give them. When you touch others, it tells them that it's okay for them to touch you. It communicates to them that you see value in them, and they will respond to you in the same way. What you give, you will always get back.

And you never know what effect you might have on someone. One teacher was speaking about the power of touch in his college classroom and, in the course of his lecture, he happened to demonstrate by touching the cheek of a young lady in the first row. She immediately burst into tears. When the teacher apologized and asked the student why she had responded so dramatically, she explained that he had touched the side of her face that had been marked since birth with a port wine stain, a large purplish birthmark. She said, "No one has ever touched it before." Her life had passed without anyone ever communicating acceptance of her birthmark by the simple act of touch. Instead, she had always felt that it must be so hideous and grotesque that no one could ever accept it or her. The teacher allowed her a few moments to understand what had happened, then with her permission, asked the entire class, one by one, to come and touch her face. Her life was changed forever by a simple touch.

Listen to Music. Music nourishes the soul. It reaches places in your being that consciousness cannot find. It allows for emotional response not directed at any particular problem in life so that you can feel its meaning without the threat of having to solve something. Music tells you that the problems you face are not yours alone but are common to humanity. It expands your connection to the human race. It doesn't matter what style of music you prefer. All that matters is that you allow it to speak to you and gain from it the insight it offers, though you probably won't be able to put it into words. If you really don't know much about music, it may take a while for you to learn the language that music speaks, but it is worth the effort. If you are not getting much out of the music you listen you, try something different. Some music is intended to simply be an expression of teenage angst. That's great if you are an angry teenager. There is also music meant for relaxation or meditation. Then there is the powerful drama of opera. It all has its place. Listen to music that moves you.

Get a massage. While this seems like a physical therapy, it does wonders for the emotions. It creates peace and relaxation like nothing else and releases emotional tension built up in the muscles. Often we let our worries and stresses just tie us up in knots. We end up holding emotional energy in our neck and shoulder muscles, causing them to tighten, stiffen, and cut off both blood flow and nerve signals. We don't even realize it, except for the headache that we just can't beat, and maybe some numbness in our hands and forearms. As we do all of that, toxins are building up in those muscles and being trapped. A good massage therapist (not just a skin rubber) will release those tension points and release the related points that you would never imagine are connected. Honestly, you may walk out feeling like you have been beat up. But the next day you will feel great. P.S.: When they tell you to drink a lot of water afterward, they mean it. If you don't flush the toxins out once they are released, you can get sick.

Laugh—out loud, long and hard. We are seeking balance. The worse you feel, the more you need a good laugh. It gets oxygen flowing; it shakes up your liver; it releases endorphins in your brain; it releases tension. Besides all that, once you start laughing, you start to put life in perspective, and you might even learn to laugh at yourself. If you need something to laugh at, the video stores will be glad to help and have collected seventy years' worth of great comedy. The Marx Brothers, Mel Brooks, and Jerry Lewis may be funnier than you remember. Cary Grant did some pretty great stuff, too, like *Bringing Up Baby* and *Arsenic and Old Lace*. Another source is *Reader's Digest*, which even has a section titled "Laughter Is the Best Medicine." One of my favorite sources is a list of actual statements made on accident reports turned in to insurance companies:

- The guy was all over the road: I had to swerve a number of times before I finally hit him.
- I pulled away from the side of the road, glanced at my mother-in-law, and headed over the embankment.
- The telephone pole was approaching fast. I was attempting to swerve out of its path when it struck the front end of my car.
- The pedestrian had no idea which direction to go, so I ran over him.

There is also a list of statements from church bulletins that don't quite say what was intended:

- Tuesday at 7:00 P.M. there will be an invitation to an ice cream social. All ladies giving milk, please come early.
- Wednesday the Ladies Literary Society will meet and Mrs. Lacey will sing "Put Me in My Little Bed," accompanied by the Reverend.

- This Sunday, being Easter, we will ask Mrs. Daley to come forward and lay an egg on the altar.

In my early years in medicine, my hospital staff responsibilities required time spent as a part of the Medical Records Committee. Here are some quotes from medical records over the years that have made me laugh. I bet you will, too!

- Patient has chest pain if she lies on her left side for over a year.
- On the second day the knee was better and on the third day it had completely disappeared.
- She has had no rigors or shaking chills, but her husband states she was very hot in bed last night.
- The patient has been depressed ever since she began seeing me in 1993.
- Patient was released to outpatient department without dressing.
- The patient is tearful and crying constantly. .She also appears to be depressed.
- Discharge status: Alive but without permission.
- The patient will need disposition, and therefore we will get Dr. Blank to dispose of him.
- Healthy appearing, decrepit 69-year-old male, mentally alert but forgetful.
- The patient refused an autopsy.
- The patient expired on the floor uneventfully.
- Patient has left his white blood cells at another hospital.
- The patient's past medical history has been remarkably insignificant with only a forty-pound weight gain in the past three days.
- She slipped on the ice and apparently her legs went in separate directions in early December.
- The patient experienced sudden onset of severe shortness of breath with a picture of acute pulmonary edema at home while having sex which gradually deteriorated in the emergency room.

- The patient had waffles for breakfast and anorexia for lunch.
- Between you and me, we ought to be able to get this lady pregnant.
- She is numb from her toes down.
- While in the ER, she was examined, X-rated, and sent home.
- Occasional, constant, infrequent headaches.
- When she fainted, her eyes rolled around the room.
- Rectal exam revealed a normal-size thyroid.
- She stated that she had been constipated for most of her life until 1995 when she got a divorce.
- The patient lives at home with his mother, father, and pet turtle, who is presently enrolled in day care three times a week.
- Bleeding started in the rectal area and continued all the way to Los Angeles.
- Exam of genitalia reveals that he is circus sized.
- Exam of genitalia was completely negative except for the right foot.
- The lab test indicated abnormal lover function.
- The patient was to have a bowel resection. However, he took a job as a stockbroker instead.
- Skin: Somewhat pale but present.
- The pelvic examination will be done later on the floor.
- Admitted in error.
- Patient was seen in consultation by Dr. .Blank, who felt we should sit on the abdomen and I agree.
- Large brown stool ambulating in the hall.
- Patient has two teenage children but no other abnormalities.
- Dr. Blank is watching his prostate.
- If he squeezes the back of his neck for four or five years, it comes and goes.

Realize that you can be as miserable as you want to be. Life is difficult. Those who expect that life should be easy end up whining and complaining how they were singled out for affliction, as if no one else knew what trouble was. Once you accept the fact that life is difficult, you are on the road to taking responsibility for your life. The worst thing you can do is start thinking of yourself as a victim. The difficulties you face in life are what they are, no more and no less. It is up to you to decide whether to be miserable about it or not. Pain is inevitable; misery is optional.

Tim Hansel broke his back in a rock-climbing accident. After years of treatment, living with constant pain, and a plethora of doctors, he went to one specialist who was touted as the final authority on his situation. He writes of their meeting in his book, *You Gotta Keep Dancin'*:

> "You'd like to know what I can do for you medically. Correct?"
> "Yes."
> "Not a darn thing."
>
> I was taken aback, but somehow, the way he said it, it didn't seem like a negative remark.
>
> "What do you suggest I do?"
> "Son, listen to me carefully. The damage has been done. The worst is over. You will have to live with pain, but that's a small price to pay for life. My recommendation is that you live your life as fully and richly as possible, . . . bite the bullet and live to be a hundred, . . ."
> "Does this mean the ball is in my court? From here on, it's up to me?"
> "Absolutely. The choice is yours."[66]

From that moment, Tim Hansel realized that he was in control of his health and his life, not the doctors, not the pain. Whatever was to become of him was his choice.

You have a choice, too. You can live in misery or you can enjoy life, even when it is difficult. You can be lonely or you can make friends. You can whine that no one cares about you or you can make yourself touchable. You can grumble, complain, snipe, and scoff, or you can laugh. The choice is yours. You can be as miserable as you want to be *or* you can bite the bullet and live to be a hundred.

Good Things for the Spirit

The best definition of spirituality is: seeking to know where you fit in with everything. Man, being created in God's (Spirit) image, is a spirit, residing in a body, possessing a soul. It is the absolute unity of these three dimensions that makes us human. The body relates us to the physical world, both to learn from it and to fashion it to meet our needs. The soul relates our physical aspects to our immaterial aspects, acting as an interface between the body and the mind. The spirit is that part of us that transcends all that we are physically and emotionally so that we are irreducible. There is always something beyond, something more. The spirit relates man to ideas, values, virtues, community, and to God.

As far as human functions, the mind and the volition are related to the spirit. In both of these functions, we reach beyond ourselves. Through the mind, we gain knowledge and, to a certain extent, become that which we know, expanding ourselves in the process. Through the will, we choose to love, extending ourselves beyond the boundaries of who "I" am to become "we." It is when we seek knowledge and seek to extend ourselves to others that we are spiritual, living in our spirits. When we cease to seek or to extend, we shrink ourselves and our spirit dies.

There is only one good thing that the spirit needs to maintain balance. It is the one and only thing that the mind craves: Truth. In turn, the will acts upon that which the mind perceives to be Truth to reach its proper object: Good. These functions can only be in balance when they are directed toward their proper object: Truth. When the mind is directed toward falsehood, it becomes obsessed, it rationalizes, it distorts reality, and it represses anything that might point it toward the Truth. When the mind is misdirected in this way, the will may choose a lesser Good, even when a greater Good is available (like choosing adultery rather than fidelity). In some cases, the will chooses harmful, self-destructive behaviors because the mind's concept of the Truth is distorted, as in the case of addictions. False beliefs can destroy our self-image, our relationships, our careers, and our health. It is when we seek Truth that we prosper and grow. It is when we choose what is truly Good that our relationships work, even our relationship with ourselves. Only then can the spirit of man be rightly related to all things; that is, the person *knows* where he fits in and he acts appropriately.

Balance is maintained by acknowledging that there is a power greater than us which has created us. Indeed, as God declares, we are "fearfully and wonderfully made." Next, we must learnthat we are *not* God. He is infinitely good, all-knowing, and all-powerful. We have some good, some knowledge, and some power, but spend most of our lives dealing with the consequences of the harm we have caused ourselves and others out of ignorance and inability to exercise self-control. If these things are true, then the next step is to ask for help. We cannot find Truth by ourselves, nor can we act on it to correct our relationships. We need enlightenment, we need guidance, and we need help to change. Until we are in this process of changing to conform our thoughts and actions to the Truth, we are out of balance.

Notice that this is a process, not a product. You will never have all Truth locked up so that there is nothing left to seek, nor will your will so perfectly conform to it that you have reached perfection. It does not take perfection to be spiritual. You simply have to be on the journey, the process toward perfection. It takes a willingness to seek honestly and to change readily. Seek and you will find!

What does this have to do with health? False beliefs lead to bad choices. This in turn corrupts our relationships with everyone around us, including ourselves. We then must live with the consequences of all those choices in an atmosphere of emotional stress, guilt, and shame. That directly effects our emotional state, which leads to chemical changes in our brains and our bodies that result in physical sickness. That makes a direct correlation between spiritual health and physical health, a correlation recognized by Dr. Ornish, who made daily meditation another central feature in his program.

The way to spiritual health is no secret. It will require prayer, meditation, and time spent in study and in reflection. In short, it will require discipline. We will not find the answers within ourselves, as many have said. We need input from those who have trodden this path before us and attained wisdom. So we discipline ourselves to read. We will not understand what we have read if we do not spend time in contemplation of the hope that Truth brings us, so we discipline ourselves to meditate. In meditation, we become convinced of the Truth how we must change to live in it. But to utilize that Truth, to truly choose Good, we need help, desperately. So we ask for help; we pray. "And it *shall* be given unto you." This is good news!

It will also require service to others, for we do not know who we are until we reach outside of ourselves and learn to give. That is the goal of spirituality: to extend and expand ourselves, to become more than we have ever been before. But first it will require the willingness to take responsibility for our lives and change. The word "repent" comes from Latin roots which mean "to think again." We must be willing to think again about our lives, and think differently, so that we may change the course of our futures. This is true of our spiritual health, our emotional health, and our physical health. Confronting ourselves with the Truth will require that we think again about the course that we want to take. We can take a path that leads to degeneration and death, or we can choose a way that leads to Truth, and ultimately to health and to life.

Attaining wholeness, and then maintaining it, is a life-long endeavor. There is never a quick fix, no simple remedy, and no magic solution. Remember, all the antioxidants in the world won't help if your spirit is being torn apart by false beliefs and your soul is being crushed by loneliness. Those forces are more powerful and pervasive than dangerous free radicals, and just as deadly. Likewise, if you have read this whole book, and don't do anything to change your antioxidant status, how will that help you find Life? We must take responsibility for our bodies, for our souls, and for our spirits.

You are a whole, not merely a bunch of parts. Treat yourself as a whole, and you can achieve wholeness. The tragedy of oxidative stress is that it eats away at us all over our bodies and steals our wholeness. The tragedy of bad choices is that they do the same thing to our souls and spirits. Death enters in either way, for death comes to the whole man.

My wish for you is that you prosper in all respects. Seek wisdom, that rare ability to learn the Truth and to live in its light. Seek love, that rare ability to accept and be accepted. And believe that strength, vitality, youthfulness, and longevity can be yours by giving your body the good things that it needs to overcome the scourge of aging.

Time is inevitable; degenerative disease is not!

Choose Life, and Life can be yours; and you can have it abundantly.

Endnotes

1. B. M. Babior, *New England Journal of Medicine* 1978.
2. J. Kedziora, *Journal of Free Radical Biology and Medicine* 1988.
3. "Third National Health and Nutrition Examination Survey," *JAMA* Apr. 24, 1966; 275.
   4 F. J. Kelly et al., *Respiratory Medicine* 1995; 89: 647–656.
5. Dr. Michael Murray, *Encyclopedia of Natural Medicine*, revised second edition, Prima Publishers (1998).
6. Ibid.
7. Ibid.
8. H. I. Chopra et al. (GREPO, Universite Joseph Fourier, La Trouche, France), "Effect of increased fruit and vegetable intake on the susceptibility of lipoprotein to oxidation in smokers," *Eur J Clin Nutr* Sept. 1997; 51 (9): 601–606.
9. H. N. Hodis et al., "Serial Coronary Angiographic Evidence that Antioxidant Vitamin Intake Reduces Progression of Coronary Artery Atherosclerosis," *JAMA* 1995; 73: 1849–1854.
10. J. A. Vinson et al., "In Vitro and In Vivo Reduction of Erythrocyte Sorbitol by Ascorbic Acid," *Diabetes* 1989; 38: 1036–1041.
11. J. T. Salonen et al., "Increased Risk of Non Insulin Diabetes Mellitus and Low Plasma Vitamin E Concentrations: A Four-Year Follow-Up Study in Men," *British Medical Journal* 1995; 311: 1124–1127.
12. A. D. Moordian and J. E. Morley, "Micronutrient Status in Diabetes Mellitus," *American Journal of Clinical Nutrition* 1987; 45: 877–895.
13. W. R. Markesbery, "Oxidative Stress Hypothesis in Alzheimer's Disease," *Free Radical Biol Med* 1997; 23: 134–147.
14. H. A. Weinreb, "Fingerprint Patterns in Alheimer's Disease," *Arch Neurol* 1985; 42: 50–54.
15. T. Cenacchi et al., *Journal of Aging* 1993; 5: 123–133.
16. P. L. LeBars et al., "A Placebo-Controlled Double-Blind Random-ized Trial of an Extract of Gingko Biloba for Dementia," *JAMA* 1997; 278: 1327–1332.
17. "Taming Oxygen's Wild Side: How Antioxidants Guard Your Health," Tapestry Press (1988), p. 9.

18. G. Ravaglia, P. Forti et al., *Journal of the American Geriatric Society* Oct. 1997: 1196–1202.

19. Buffington et al., *American Journal of Medical Science* Nov. 1993: 320–324.

20. Araghi-Niknam et al., *Proc Soc Exp Biol Med* Dec. 1997: 386–391.

21. M. A. Lane et al., *Journal of Clinical Endocrinology Metabolism* July 1997: 2093–2096.

22. Benjamin Lau, M.D., *Garlic and You: The Modern Medicine*, Apple Publishing Co. (1997).

23. Ibid.

24. Ibid.

25. Robert Crayhon, *Robert Crayhon's Nutrition Made Simple*, M. Evans and Company: New York (1994).

26. Notes from Wakunaga of America Company.

27. Leo Galland, M.D., *The Four Pillars of Healing,* Random House: New York (1997), p. 197.

28. Ibid, p. 137

29. Earl Mindell and Virginia Hopkins, *Dr. Earl Mindell's What You Should Know About the Super Antioxidant Miracle*, Keats(1996).

30. Ibid.

31. T. T. Yang and M. W. Koo, "Hypocholesterolemic effects of Chinese tea," *Pharmacology Resources* June 1997: 505–12.

32. Donald J. Brown, *Herbs for Health* Sept.–Oct. 1997.

33. Ibid.

34. Daniel B. Mowrey, *The Scientific Validation of Herbal Medicine* (1986).

35. Pierre Le Bars, Martin Katz et al., "A Placebo-Controlled, Double-Blind, Randomized Trial of an Extract of Ginkgo Biloba for Dementia," *JAMA* Oct. 22/29, 1997; 278 (16): 1327.

36. Donald J. Brown, *Herbs for Health* Sept.–Oct. 1997.

37. Ibid.

38. H. Hikino et al., "The Antihepatotoxic Actions of Flavonolignans from Silybum marianum Fruits," *Planta Medica* 1984; 50: 248–50.

39. A. Valenzuela et al., *Planta Medica* 55 1989; 50: 420–422.

40. G. Buzzelli et al., "A Pilot Study on the Liver Protective Effect of Silybin-Phosphatidylcholine Complex (IdB1016) in Chronic Active Hepatitis," *International Journal of Clinical Pharmacology, Therapeutics, and Toxicology* 1993; 31: 456–460.

41. Walter Pierpaoli and William Regelson with Carol Colman, *The Melatonin Miracle*, Simon & Shuster: New York (1995), pp. 34–35.

42. Ibid. pp. 51, 56.
43. Steven J. Bock, M.D., and Michael Boyette, *Stay Young the Melatonin Way*, Penguin Books: New York (1996), p. 65.
44. Michael T. Murray, N.D., *5-HTP: The Natural Way to Overcome Depression, Obesity, and Insomnia*, Bantam Books: New York (1998).
45. A. Castano et al., "Changes in the turnover of monoamines in prefrontal cortex of rats fed on vitamin E - deficient diet." *Journal of Neurochemistry* 1992; 58: 1889–95
46. Michael T. Murray, N.D., *5-HTP: The Natural Way to Overcome Depression, Obesity, and Insomnia* Bantam Books: New York (1998).
47. James F. Balch, Jr., MD., *Prescription for Nutritional Healing,* Avery Publishing Company: New York.
48. Ibid.
49. Ibid.
50. Dr. Richard Passwater, "Important AIDS Discovery Explains the Importance of Selenium: An Interview with Will Taylor, Ph.D." *Whole Foods Magazine.*
51. Ibid.
52. *Science News* 151:239 (April 19, 1997).
53. *Healing Yourself with Food* Rodale Press: Emmaus, Penn (1995).
54. Earl Mindell and Virginia Hopkins, *Dr. Earl Mindell's What You Should know About the Super Antioxidant Miracle*, Keats (1996)
55. Ibid.
56. Ibid.
57. Ibid.
58. Ibid.
59. Ibid.
60. Ibid.
61. Ibid.
62. Ibid.
63. Ibid.
64. Elaine Conner, M.D., and Matthew Grisham, M.D., *Nutrition* 1996; 2: 274–277.
65. I. Hininger et al., *European Journal of Clinical Nutrition* 1997; 51: 01–606.
66. Tim Hansel, *You Gotta Keep Dancin'*, David C. Cook Publishing (1985), pp. 66–67.

Acknowledgments

Many would say that a surgeon's occupation is the most difficult thing. I would disagree, declaring that writing a book of nonfiction and vital to the life and health of people is far more agonizing. I would first like to thank my wife, Dr. Robin Young-Balch, for her persistence and patience in dealing with the author in the preparation of this book. Without her, this work would not have been possible.

To my assistant, Ron Brooks, a talented writer in his own right, and to Steve Pascal, a beginner, yet extremely hard worker, I thank you.

And how would this all have been accomplished without my "right hand," Ms. Eva Martin, whose diligence and helpful direction played a significant role in the completion of this manuscript.

And finally, to Mr. George de Kay, Publisher of M. Evans and Company, and Nancy Hancock, Editor, who worked so many long hours, along with those behind the scenes at M. Evans.

Last, but not least, my good friend and co-worker, Kevin Miller, who initiated this entire project and continued to encourage me until the work was finished.

I thank you all.

Glossary

adaptogen—A substance that builds resistance to stress by strengthening the immune system, nervous system, and/or glandular system.* A substance, usually an herb, that produces suitable adjustments in the body. They tend to normalize body functions and when the job is complete, they are eliminated or incorporated into the body without side effects. Some adaptogens are: garlic, ginseng, echinacea, ginkgo biloba, golden seal, and Pau d'Arc.

aerobic metabolism—Living and growing in the presence of oxygen by necessity.

alkaloid—One of a large group of nitrogen-containing alkaline substances found in plants; usually very bitter and pharmacologically active.*

allergen—A substance that provokes an allergic response.

allergy—An inappropriate response by the immune system to a normally harmless substance. Allergies can affect any of the body's tissues.

amino acids—The building blocks of proteins, which are synthesized by living cells or are obtained as essential components of the diet.*

anoxia—Lack of oxygen in a cell, tissue, or organ.*

antibiotic—A substance produced by a microorganism that is capable of killing or inhibiting the growth of bacteria or other microorganisms.*

* Taken from *Herbs for Health* magazine, September/October 1997, pp. 21, 23.

antibody—A protein molecule made by the immune system that is designed to intercept and neutralize a specific invading organism or other foreign substance.

antigen—A substance that can elicit the formation of an antibody when introduced into the body.

antihistamine—A substance that interferes with the action of histamines by binding to histamine receptors in various body tissues.

antioxidant—A compound that prevents cell damage by free radicals or oxidation; a compound, vitamin, or enzyme that blocks or inhibits destructive oxidation reaction and free radicals. Examples include: vitamins A, C, and E; the minerals selenium and germanium; the enzymes catalase, superoxide dismutase (SOD), Co-enzyme Q-10, and some amino acids, etc.* A compound or enzyme opposing oxidant action.

antioxidant adaptation—Adjustments by the antioxidant defenses to compensate for increased oxidative stress to cells, tissues, or organs.

arteriosclerosis—A circulatory disorder characterized by thickening and stiffening of the walls of large and medium-sized arteries, ultimately impeding circulation.

atherosclerosis—The most common type of arteriosclerosis, caused by the accumulation of fatty deposits in the inner linings of the arteries.

autoimmune disorder—Any condition in which the immune system reacts inappropriately to the body's own tissues and attacks them. This causes damage or interference with normal functioning. Examples include: diabetes, multiple sclerosis, rheumatoid arthritis, and systemic lupus erythematosus.

benign—Literally means "harmless," referring to cells that grow in an inappropriate location but that do not invade (not cancerous or malignant).

beta-carotene—A pigment found in milk, some yellow and dark green vegetables such as broccoli, spinach, and carrots, and in fruits such as cantaloupes, peaches, and apricots. The body converts beta-carotene to vitamin A, which is essential for normal eyesight, healthy tissue, a strong immune system, and bone development.* A substance the body uses to make pro-vitamin A, a carotenoid.

bioflavonoid—Any of the flavonoids (a class of substances widely found in flowers, leaves, and fruits) with biological activity in

mammals.* A group of biologically active flavonoids sometimes referred to as vitamin P.

blood-brain barrier—A mechanism involving the capillaries and
other cells of the brain that keeps many substances from passing out of the bloodstream into the brain tissue.

capillaries—The tiniest of blood vessels, generally one cell thick,
they allow the exchange of nutrients and wastes between the
bloodstream and the body's cells.

carbohydrates—Many organic substances, almost all of plant origin, that are composed of carbon, hydrogen, and oxygen and
serve as the major source of energy in the diet (a complex
sugar).

carcinogen—A substance causing cellular transformation and malignancy; an agent capable of causing cancer.* A substance
causing nepotistic transformation and eventually malignancy
(cancer); An agent that is capable of inducing cancerous
changes in cells and/or tissues.

cardiac—Pertaining to the heart.

cholesterol—A crystlym substance that is soluble in fats and that
is produced by all vertebrates. It is a necessary constitution of
cell membranes, and facilitates the transport and absorption
of fatty acids.

chemotherapy—The treatment of disease by chemical agents.*

coenzyme—A molecule that works with an enzyme to enable the
enzyme to perform its function in the body. Coenzymes are
necessary in the utilization of vitamins and minerals.

complex carbohydrates—A type of carbohydrate that, owing to
its chemical structure, releases its sugar into the blood slowly
and also provides fiber. The carbohydrates in starches and
fiber are complex and are also called polysaccharides.

dementia—Mental deterioration due to organic causes.*

detoxification—The process of reducing the build up of various
poisonous substances in the body.

detoxicative biotransformation—The biochemical processing of
a compound that results in its eventual decreased toxicity.

DHEA—Dehydroepiandrosterone, a natural hormone manufactured by the adrenal gland. It is the major androgen precursor
in females.*

diabetes mellitus—A chronic disorder in which the body is unable to utilize carbohydrates properly, either because of a lack

of the hormone insulin (Type I diabetes) or because of inability to use insulin (Type II diabetes).*

DNA (deoxyribonucleic acid)—The substance in the cell nucleus that genetically contains the cell's genetic blueprint determining the type of life form into which a cell will develop.

endocrine system—A system of ductless glands, including the thyroid, thymus, pituitary, and adrenal, as well as the panceas, ovaries, and testes, whose secretions, released directly into the bloodstream, have a critical impact on physiological activity .*

endorphin—One of a number of natural hormonelike substances found primarily in the brain. One function of endorphins is to suppress the sensation of pain, which they do by binding to opiate receptors in the brain.

enzyme—One of many specific proteins that initiate or speed chemical reactions in the body.

essential fatty acids (EFAs)—Any fatty acid that cannot be synthesized by the body and must be obtained from dietary sources.*

fats—Lipids; easily stored in the body and important as a source of fuel and to cell structure.*

free radicals—An atom or group of atoms that is highly reactive because it has at least one unpaired electron. Because they join so readily with other compounds, free radicals can attack cells and can cause great damage in the body. Free radical damage plays a role in virtually every major chronic disease and is thought to be a driving force of human aging. Free radicals form in heated fats and oils and as a result of exposure to atmospheric radiation and environmental pollutants, etc. Antioxidants counteract free radicals.*

free radical quencher and scavenger—A molecule able to react with and thereby neutralize a free radical, often becoming oxidized in the process; a substance that removes or destroys free radicals.

ginsenosides—Active compounds (eleven major, nineteen minor) found only in ginseng that are responsible for its health benefits.*

glucose—The most common simple sugar in the body and the main source of energy for humans.*

glycogen—The body's main carbohydrate reserve.*

heavy metal—A metallic element such as arsenic, cadmium, lead, and mercury.

homeostasis—Processes which maintain equilibrium in living systems.

hormone—One of numerous essential substances produced by the endocrine glands that regulate many bodily functions.

hydrogenation—A chemical process used to turn liquid oils into a more solid form by bombarding the oil molecules with hydrogen atoms. Hydrogenation destroys the nutritional value of the oil and also results in the formation of trans fatty acids, altered fatty acid molecules that do not occur in nature and can be quiet harmful.

hypertension—High blood pressure.*

hypoxia—A lowered tissue oxygen tension from ischemia or anemia.

immune suppression—The impairment of immune response capacities.

immune system—A complex system that depends on the interaction of many different organs, cells, and proteins. Its chief function is to identify and eliminate foreign substances such as harmful bacteria that have invaded the body. The liver, spleen, thymus, bone marrow, and lymphatic system all play vital roles in the proper functioning of the immune system.

immunity—The condition of being able to resist and overcome disease or infection. Simply, immunity means freedom from disease.

immuno-deficiency—A defect in the functioning of the immune system. It can be inherited or acquired, reversible or permanent. Immuno-deficiency renders the body more susceptible to illness of every type, especially infectious illnesses.

immunology—The branch of medical science that deals with the functioning of the immune system.

immuno-therapy—The treatment of disease by using techniques that stimulate or strengthen the immune system.

inflammation—The sequence of homeostatic reactions evoked from affected tissues in response to injury; usually resulting in removal or destruction of the offending agent.

in vitro—Meaning under artificial conditions.

in vivo—Meaning in the living state.

ischemia—The interruption or impairment of blood flow to some part of an organ or tissue.

lipid peroxidation—The incorporation of oxygen into lipids (usually in cellular membranes) with cross linking and eventual destruction of the lipids.

lipoprotein—A type of protein molecule that incorporates a lipid.

Lipoproteins act as agents of lipid transport in the lymph and blood.

lipotropic—Any of a number of substances that can help to prevent the accumulation of abnormal amounts of fat in the liver, control blood sugar levels, and enhance fat and carbohydrate metabolism. Lipotropics include choline, inositol, methionine, and L-carnitine.

lymph—A clear liquid derived from blood plasma that circulates throughout the body, that is collected from the tissues, and that flows through the lymphatic vessels, eventually returning to the blood circulation. Its primary function is to nourish tissue cells and return waste matter into the bloodstream.

lymph nodes—Organs located along the lymphatic vessels that act as filters, trapping and removing foreign material. Within the lymph nodes are lymphocytes, immune cells that develop the capacity to seek out and destroy specific foreign agents.

lymphocyte—A type of white blood cell found in lymph, blood, and other specialized tissues such s the bone marrow and tonsils. There are several different categories of lymphocytes. These are designated as B-lymphocytes and T-lymphocytes. Also there are non-B and non-T type lymphocytes called null lymphocytes. These cells are crucial components of the immune system. B-lymphocytes are primarily responsible for antibody production, whereas the T-lymphocytes are involved in indirect attack against an invading organism.

malignant—A word that literally means "evil." It generally refers to cells or groups of cells that are cancerous and likely to spread (metastasize).

membrane—A continuous three-dimensional assembly of proteins and fats. A "work surface" for facilitating metabolic reactions and creating functional components within the cell.

membrane transport pumps—Enzymes that transport molecules across membranes that ensures their differential distribution and maintains distinguished functional compartments in the cell.

metabolism—The physical and chemical processes necessary to sustain life, including the production of cellular energy, the synthesis of important biological substances, and the degradation of various compounds.

metabolite—A substance produced as a result of a metabolic process.

neoplasia—Unregulated growth.

nutraceutical—A food or nutrient-based product or supplement designed and/or used for a specific clinical and/or therapeutic purpose.

oxidant—A compound that tends to oxidize other molecules by stealing electrons from them.

oxidation—The removal of an electron from an atom or molecule; chemical reaction in which oxygen reacts with another substance, resulting in a chemical transformation. Many oxidation reactions result in some type of deterioration or spoilage.

oxidative stress—Any action that increases oxidative potential in a living system or reduces antioxidant defenses.

peroxidation—A propagative, oxidative breakdown of fatty acids in cell membranes.

peroxidative cross-linking—An abnormal atom-to-atom bonding within or between biomolecules as a result of lipid peroxidation.

phagocyte—A cell capable of ingesting bacteria or other foreign particles. Once captured, they are usually killed with the help of activated oxygen species.

phytochemical—Any one of many substances present in fruits and vegetables that have various health-producing properties. Some phytochemicals appear to protect against cancer and other degenerative diseases.

prostaglandins—Hormonelike substances that reduce inflammation and pain, and help regulate blood pressure, blood clotting, allergic response, and heart, kidney, and gastrointestinal function.* Locally acting hormones and inflammatory mediators formed by fatty acid peroxidation.

protein—Complex substances, composed of amino acids, that serve as enzymes, structural elements, and hormones. Proteins are involved in many activities throughout the body, including oxygen transport, muscle contraction, and electron transport.* Any of many complex nitrogen-based organic compounds made up of different combinations of amino acids. Proteins are basic elements of all animal and vegetable tissues. Biological substances, such as hormones and enzymes, are composed of protein. The body makes specific proteins for growth, repair, and other functions from amino acids that are either extracted from dietary protein or manufactured from other amino acids.

saturated fats—Lipids that are usually solid at room temperature and tend to raise total blood cholesterol levels.*

synergy—An interaction between two or more substances in which their combined action is greater than their individual actions.

toxicity—The quality of being poisonous. Toxicity reactions in the body impair bodily functions and/or damage cells.

toxin—A poison that impairs the health and functioning of the body.

virus—A disease-causing agent, regarded as either an extremely simple microorganism or an extremely complex molecule, that can grow and reproduce only in living cells of plants, humans, or animals.*

vitamin—One of approximately fifteen organic substances that are essential in small quantities for life and health. Most vitamins cannot be manufactured by the body and so need to be supplied in the diet.

xenobiotic (foreign compound)—A substance not normally found in living systems.

Food Additives

Antioxidants

Antioxidants stop food from going rancid and protect fat-soluble vitamins from the harmful effects of oxidation

L-ascorbin acid—fruit drinks; also used to improve flour and bread dough

Sodium L—ascorbate

Calcium L—ascorbate

6-0-Palmitoyl-L-ascorbic Acid (ascorbyl palmitrate)—Scotch eggs

Extracts of natural origin rich in tocopherols—vegetable oils

Synthetic gamma-tocopherol

Synthetic delta-tocopherol

Propyl gallate—vegetable oils; chewing gum

Octyl gallate

Dodecyl gallate

Butylated hydroxyanisole (BHA)—soup mixes; cheese spread

Lecithins—low-fat spreads; also used as an emulsifier in chocolate

Diphenylamine

Ethoxyquin—used to prevent "scald" (a discoloration) on apples and pears

Preservatives

Preservatives protect against microbes which cause spoilage and food poisoning. They also increase storage life of foods.

Sorbic acid—soft drinks; fruit yogurt; processed cheese slices

Sodium sorbate

Potassium sorbate
Calcium sorbate—frozen pizza; flour confectionery
Benzoic acid
Sodium benzoate
Potassium benzoate
Calcium benzoate
Ethyl 4-hydroxybenzoate (ethyl para-hydroxybenzoate)
Ethyl 4-hydroxybenzoate, sodium salt (sodium ethyl para-hydroxybenzoate)
Propyl 4-hydroxybenzoate (propyl para-hydroxybenzoate)
Propyl 4-hydroxybenzoate, sodium salt (sodium propyl para-hydroxybenzoate)
Methyl 4-hydroxybenzoate (methyl para-hydroxybenzoate)
Methyl 4-hydroxybenzoate, sodium salt (sodium methyl para-hydroxybenzoate)—beer; jam; salad cream; soft drinks; fruit pulp; fruit-based pie fillings; marinated herring and mackerel
Sulphur dioxide
Sodium sulphite
Sodium hydrogen sulphite (sodium bisulphite)
Sodium metabisulphite
Potassium metabisulphite
Calcium sulphite
Calcium hydrogen sulphite (calcium bisulphite)—dried fruit; dehydrated vegetables; fruit juices and syrups; sausages; fruit-based dairy desserts; cider; beer; wine; also used to prevent browning of raw peeled potatoes and to condition biscuit doughs
Potassium bisulphite—wines
Biphenyl (diphenyl)
2-Hydroxybiphenyl (orthophenylphenol)
Sodium biphenyl-2-yl oxide (sodium orthophenylphenate)—surface treatment of citrus fruit
2-(Thiazol-4-yl) benzimidazole (thiabendazole)—surface treatment of bananas
Nisin—cheese; clotted cream
Hexamine (hexamethylenetetramine)—marinated herring and mackerel
Potassium nitrite
Sodium nitrite
Sodium nitrate

Potassium nitrate—bacon; ham; cured meats; corned beef; some cheeses
Propionic acid
Sodium propionate
Calcium propionate
Potassium propionate—bread and flour confectionery; Christmas pudding

Taken from *The Cambridge Factfinder*, Cambridge University Press, (1994), pp. 134-37.

Colors

Colors make food more colorful, compensate for color lost in processing.

Curcumin—flour confectionery; margarine
Riboflavin—sauces
Riboflavin-5-phosphate
Tartrazine—soft drinks
Quinoline yellow
Sunset Yellow FCF—biscuits
Cochineal—alcoholic drinks
Carmoisine—jams and preserves
Amaranth
Ponceau 4R—dessert mixes
Erythrosine BS—glace cherries
Red 2G—sausages
Patent Blue V
Indigo Carmine
Brilliant Blue FCF—canned vegetables
Chlorophyll
Copper complexes of chlorophyll and chlorophyllins
Green S—pastilles
Caramel—beer, soft drinks; sauces; gravy browning
Black PN
Carbon Black (vegetable carbon)—liquorice
Brown FK—kippers
Brown HT—chocolate cake
Alpha-carotene, beta-carotene, gamma-carotene—margarine; soft drinks

Annatto, bixin, norbixin—crisps / potato chips
Capsanthin, capsorubin
Beta-apo-i-carotenal
Ethyl ester of beta-apo-8-carotenoid acid
Flavoxanthin
Lutein
Cryptoxanthin
Rubixanthin
Violaxanthin
Rhodoxanthin
Canthaxanthin
Beetroot Red (betanin)—ice cream; liquorice
Anthocyanins—yogurt
Titanium dixoide—sweets
Iron oxides, iron hydroxides
Aluminum
Silver
Gold—cake decorations
Pigment Rubine (lithol rubine BK)
Methyl violet—used for the surface marking of raw or unprocessed meat
Paprika—canned vegetables
Tumeric—soup

Taken from *The Cambridge Factfinder*, Cambridge University Press, (1994), pp. 134–37.

Sweeteners

There are two types of sweeteners: intense sweeteners and bulk sweeteners. Intense sweeteners have a sweetness many times that of sugar and are therefore used at very low levels. They are marked with * in the following list. Bulk sweeteners have about the same sweetness as sugar and are used at the same sort of levels as sugar.

*Acesulfame potassium—canned foods; soft drinks; table-top sweeteners
*Aspartame—soft drinks; yogurts; dessert and drink mixes; sweetening tablets
Hydrogenated glucose syrup
Isomalt

Lactitol

Mannitol—sugar-free confectionery

*Saccharin

*Sodium saccharin

*calcium saccharin—soft drinks; cider; sweetening tablets; table-top sweeteners

Sorbitol, sorbitol syrup—sugar-free confectionery; jams for diabetics

*Thaumatin—table-top sweeteners; yogurt

Xylitol—sugar-free chewing gum

Taken from *The Cambridge Factfinder*, Cambridge University Press, (1994), pp. 134–37.

Emulsifiers and Stabilizers

Emulsifiers and Stabilizers enable oils and fats to mix with water in foods; add to smoothness and creaminess of texture; and retard staling in baked goods going stale.

Alginic acid—ice-cream; soft cheese

Sodium alginate—cake mixes

Potassium alginate

Ammonium alginate

Calcium alginate

Propane-1,2-diol alginate (propylene glycol alginate)—salad dressings; cottage cheese

Agar—ice-cream

Carrageenan—quick-setting jelly mixes; milk shakes

Locust bean gum (carob gum)—salad cream

Guar gum—packet soups and meringue mixes

Tragacanth—salad dressings; processed cheese

Gum arabic (acacia)—confectionery

Xanthan gum—sweet pickle; coleslaw

Karaya gum—sweet pickle; coleslaw

Karaya gum—soft cheese, brown sauce

Polyoxyethylene (20) sorbitan monolaurate (Polysorbate 20)

Polyoxethylene (20) sorbitan mono-oleate (Polysorbate 80)

Polyoxyethylene (20) sorbitan monopalmitate (Polysorbate 40)

Polyoxyethylene (20) sorbitan monostearate (Polysorbate 60)

Polyoxyethylene (20) sorbitan tristearate (Polysorbate 65)—bakery products; confectionery creams

(i) Pectin

(ii) Amidated pectin

Ammonium phosphatides—cocoa and chocolate products

Microcrystalline cellulose—grated cheese

Alpha-cellulose (powdered cellulose)—slimming bread

Methylcellulose—low-fat spreads

Hydroxypropylcellulose

Hydroxypropylmethylcellulose—edible ices

Ethylmethylcellulose—gateaux

Carboxymethylcellulose, sodium salt (CMC)—jelly; gateaux

Sodium, potassium and calcium salts of fatty acids—cake mixes

Mono- and di-glycerides of fatty acids—frozen deserts

Acetic acid esters of mono- and di-glycerides of fatty acids—mousse mixes

Lactic acid esters of mono- and di-glycerides of fatty acids—dessert toppings

Citric acid esters of mono- and di-glycerides of fatty acids—continental sausages

Tartaric acid esters of mono- and di-glycerides of fatty acids

Mono- and di-acetyltartaric acid esters of mono- and di-glycerides of fatty acids—bread; frozen pizza

Mixed acetic and tartaric acid esters of mono- and di-glycerides of fatty acids

Sucrose esters of fatty acids

Sucroglycerides—edible ices

Polyglycerol esters of fatty acids—cakes and gateaux

Polyglycerol esters of polycondensed fatty acids of castor oil (polyglycerol polyricinoleate)—chocolate-flavor coatings of cakes

Propane-1,2-diol esters of fatty acids—instant desserts

Sodium stearoyl-1-2-lactylate—bread; cakes; biscuits

Calcium stearoyl-1-2-lactylate—gravy granules

Stearyl tartrate

Sorbitan monostearate

Sorbitan tristearate

Sorbitan monolaurate

Sorbitan mono-oleate

Sorbitan monopalmitrate—cake mixes

Extract of quillaia—used in soft drinks to promote foam

Oxidatively polymerized soya-bean oil
Polyglycerol esters of dimerized fatty acids of soya-bean oil—emulsions used to grease bakery tins

Taken from *The Cambridge Factfinder*, Cambridge University Press, (1994), pp. 134–37.

Other

Acids, anti-caking agents, anti-foaming agents, bases, buffers, bulking agents, firming agents, flavor modifiers, flour improvers, glazing agents, humectants, liquid freezants, packaging gases, propellants, release agents, sequestrants, and solvents.

Calcium carbonate—base, firming agent, release agent, diluent; nutrient in flour
Acetic acid
Potassium acetate
Sodium hydrogen diacetate
Sodium acetate—acid/acidity regulators (buffers) used in pickles, salad cream and bread; they contribute to flavor and provide protection against mold growth
Calcium acetate—firming agent; also provides calcium which is useful in quick-set jelly mix
Lactic acid—acid/flavoring protects against mold growth; salad dressing; soft margarines
Carbon dioxide—carbonating agent/packaging gas and propellant; used in fizzy drinks
DL-malic acid, L-malic acid
Fumaric acid—acid/flavoring; used in soft drinks, sweets, biscuits, dessert mixes, and pie fillings
Sodium lactate—buffer, humectant; used in jams, preserves, sweets, flour confectionery
Potassium lactate—buffer, jams, preserves and jellies
Calcium lactate—buffer, firming agent; canned fruit, pie filling
Citric acid
Sodium dihydrogen citrate (monosodium citrate), disodium citrate, trisodium citrate
Potassium dihydrogen citrate (monopotassium citrate), tripotassium citrate

Monocalcium citrate, dicalcium citrate, tricalcium citrate—acid/ flavorings, buffers, sequestrants, emulsifying salts (calcium salts are firming agents); used in soft drinks, jams, preserves, sweets, UHT cream, processed cheese, canned fruit, dessert mixes, ice cream

L-(+)tartaric acid

Monosodium L-(+)-tartrate, disodium L-(+)-tartrate

Monopotassium L-(+)-tartrate (cream of tartar), dipotassium L- (+)-tartrate

Potassium sodium L-(+)-tartrate—acid/flavorings, buffers, emulsifying salts, sequestrants; used in soft drinks, biscuit creams and fillings, sweets, jams, dessert mixes and processed cheese

Orthophosphoric acid (phosphoric acid)—acid/flavorings; soft drinks, cocoa

Sodium dihydrogen orthophosphate, disodium hydrogen orthophosphate, trisodium orthophosphate

Potassium dihydrogen orthophosphate, dipotassium hydrogen orthophosphate, tripotassium orthophosphate—buffers, sequestrants, emulsifying salts; used in dessert mixes, non-dairy creamers, processed cheese

Calcium tetrahydrogen diorthophosphate, calcium hydrogen orthophosphate, tricalcium diorthophospate—firming agent, anti-caking agent, raising agent; cake mixes, baking powder, dessert mixes

Sodium malate, sodium hydrogen malate

Potassium malate—buffers, humectants; used in jams, sweets, cakes, biscuits

Calcium maltate; calcium hydrogen malate—firming agent in processed fruit and vegetables

Metatartaric acid—sequestrant used in wine

Adipic acid—buffer/flavoring; sweets, synthetic cream desserts

Succinic acid—buffer/flavoring; dry foods and beverage mixes

1,4-heptonolactone—acid, sequestrant; dried soups, instant desserts

Nicotinic acid—color stabilizer and nutrient; bread, flour, breakfast cereals

Triammonium citrate—buffer, emulsifying salt; processed cheese

Ammonium ferric citrate—dietary iron supplement; bread

Calcium disodium ethylenediamine-NNN'N'-tetra-acetate (calcium disodium EDTA)—sequestrant; canned shellfish

Glycerol—humectant, solvent; cake icing, confectionery

Disodium dihydrogen diphosphate, trisodium diphosphate, tetrasodium diphosphate, tetrapotassium diphosphate

Pentasodium triphosphate, pentapotassium triphosphate

Sodium polyphosphates, potassium polyphosphates—buffers, sequestrants, emulsifying salts, stabilizers, texturizers, raising agents; used in whipping cream, fish and meat products, bread, processed cheese, canned vegetables

Sodium carbonate, sodium hydrogen carbonate (bicarbonate of soda), sodium sequicarbonate

Potassium carbonate, potassium hydrogen carbonate—bases, aerating agents, diluents; used in jams, jellies, self-raising flour, wine, cocoa

Ammonium carbonate, ammonium hydrogen carbonate—buffer, aerating agent; cocoa, biscuits

Magnesium carbonate—base, anti-caking agent, wafer biscuits, icing sugar

Hydrochloric acid

Potassium chloride—gelling agent, salt substitute; table-salt replacement

Calcium chloride—firming agent in canned fruit and vegetables

Ammonium chloride—yeast food in bread

Sulphuric acid

Sodium sulphate—diluent for colors

Potassium sulphate—salt substitute

Calcium sulphate—firming agent and yeast food; bread

Magnesium sulphate—firming agent

Sodium hydroxide—base; cocoa, jams and sweets

Potassium hydroxide—base; sweets

Calcium hydroxide—firming agent; neutralizing agent; sweets

Ammonium hydroxide—diluent and solvent for food colors, base; cocoa

Magnesium hydroxide—base; sweets

Calcium oxide—base; sweets

Magnesium oxide—anti-caking agent; cocoa products

Sodium ferrocyanide

Potassium ferrocyanide—anti-caking agents in salt; crystallization aids in wine

Dicalcium diphosphate—buffer, neutralizing agent; cheese

Sodium aluminum phosphate—acid, raising agent; cake mixes,

self-raising flour, biscuits

Edible bone phosphate—anti-caking agent

Calcium polyphosphates—emulsifying salt; processed cheese

Ammonium polyphosphates—emulsifier, texturizer; frozen chicken

Silicon dioxide (silica)—anti-caking agent; skimmed milk powder, sweeteners

Calcium silicate—anti-caking agent, release agent; icing sugar, sweets

Magnesium silicate, and synthetic magnesium trisilicate—anti-caking agent; sugar confectionery

Talc—release agent; tabletted confectionery

Aluminum sodium silicate

Aluminum calcium silicate

Bentonite

Kaolin

Stearic acid—anti-caking agents

Magnesium stearate—emulsifier, release agent; confectionery

D-glucono-1,5-lactone (glucono delta-lactone)—acid, sequestrant; cake mixes, continental sausages

Sodium gluconate

Potassium gluconate—sequestrants

Calcium gluconate—buffer, firming agent, sequestrant; jams, dessert mixes

L-glutamic acid

Sodium hydrogen L-glutamate (monosodium glutamate; MSG)

Potassium hydrogen L-glutamate (monopotassium glutamate)

Calcium dihydrogen di-L-glutamate (calcium glutamate)

Guanosine 5'-disodium phosphate (sodium guanylate)

Inosine 5'-disodium phosphate (sodium inosinate)

Sodium 5'-ribonucleotide—flavor enhancers used in savory foods and snacks, soups, sauces and meat products

Maltol

Ethyl maltol—flavorings/flavor enhancers used in cakes and biscuits

Dimethylpolysiloxante—anti-foaming agent

Beeswax

Carnauba wax—glazing agents used in sugar and chocolate confectionery

Shellac—glazing agent used to wax apples

Mineral hydrocarbons—glazing/coating agent used to prevent dried fruit sticking together

Refined microcrystalline wax—release agent; chewing gum

L-cysteine hydrochloride

Chlorine

Chlorine dioxide

Azodicarbonamide—flour-treatment agents used to improve the texture of bread, cake, and biscuit doughs

Aluminum potassium sulphate—firming agent; chocolate-coated cherries

2-Aminoethanol—base; caustic lye used to peel vegetables

Ammonium dihydrogen orthophosphate; diammonium hydrogen orthophosphate—buffer, yeast food

Ammonium sulphate—yeast food

Benzoyl peroxide—bleaching agent in flour

Butyl stearate—release agent

Calcium heptonate—firming agent, sequestrant; prepared fruit and vegetables

Calcium phytate—sequestrant; wine

Dichlorodifluoromethane—propellant and liquid freezant used to freeze food by immersion

Diethyl ether—solvent

Disodium dihydrogen ethylenediamine-NNN'N'-tetra-acetate (disodium dihydrogen EDTA)—sequestrant; brandy

Ethanol (ethylalcohol)

Ethyl acetate

Glycerol mono-acetate (monoacetin)

Glycerol di-acetate (diacetin)

Glycerol tri-acetate (triacetin)—solvents used to dilute and carry food colors and flavorings

Glycine—sequestrant, buffer, nutrient

Hydrogen

Nitrogen—packaging gases

Nitrous oxide—propellant used in aerosol packs of whipped cream

Octadecylammonium acetate—anti-caking agent in yeast foods used in bread

Oxygen—packing gas

Oxystearin—sequestrant, fat crystallization inhibitor; salad cream

Polydextrose—bulking agent; reduced- and low-calorie foods

Propan-1,2-diol (propylene glycol)

Propan-2-diol (isopropyl alcohol)—solvents used to dislute col-
ors and flavorings
Sodium heptonate—sequestrant; edible oils
Spermaceti
Sperm oil—release agents
Tannic acid—flavoring, clarifying agent; beer, wine and cider

Taken from *The Cambridge Factfinder*, Cambridge University Press,
(1994), pp. 134–37.

Index

You Gotta Keep Dancin' (Hansel), 266
Yucca, 170

Zeaxanthin, 75, 128
Zinc
 and Alzheimer's disease, 77, 79
 benefits of, 214–215
 and bilberry, 183
 and cancer, 216, 218

and colds, 215–216
and diabetes, 68–69, 216, 218
dietary sources of, 69, 218–219
dosage of, 218
and Down's syndrome, 87–88
and macular degeneration, 76
malabsorption of, 77–78
and selenium, 210
Zutphen Elderly Study, 120